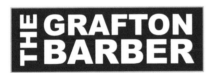

GROOMING & ETIQUETTE
FOR GENTLEMEN & THEIR SONS

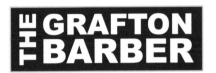

GROOMING & ETIQUETTE
FOR GENTLEMEN & THEIR SONS

CONOR & HUGH
McALLISTER

with Caitlin McBride

Foreword by
JAMES NESBITT

BLACK & WHITE PUBLISHING

First published 2018
by Black & White Publishing Ltd
Nautical House, 104 Commercial Street, Edinburgh, EH6 6NF

1 3 5 7 9 10 8 6 5 4 2   18 19 20 21

ISBN: 978 1 78530 217 6

Images on pages: 4, 13, 21, 23, 25, 29, 31, 43, 47, 48, 51, 52, 55, 63, 64, 65, 67, 70, 73, 74, 76, 80,
86, 87, 91, 93, 95, 99, 101, 103, 104(bottom), 105, 106, 107, 108, 109, 111, 116, 117, 123, 128, 131,
139, 143, 144, 145, 146 © Shutterstock.com
Images on pages: 37, 59, 125(bottom), 137 © iStock.com
Images on pages: 109, 125(top) © Alamy Stock Photo / Hero Images Inc., LightField Studios Inc.
Images on page 41 © Anthony Woods Photography
Images on pages: vi(top), 57 © Sean Cahill
Image on page vi(bottom) © Tony Gavin/INM

Illustrations on pages: 32, 33, 34, 38, 39, 60, 62, 65, 71, 81, 85, 86, 129, 141 © Shutterstock.com
Illustrations on pages: 17, 34, 44, 50, 54, 64 © iStock.com
Illustration on page 97 © Rawpixel/Freepik. Illustration on page 104(top) © Freepik.

All other images © Conor McAllister and Hugh McAllister

Page 119: Michael Phelps quote, *Business Insider*, 10.08.2016.
Page 128: quote from Steve Jobs' Commencement Address, *Stanford News*, 14.06.2005.
Page 137: Walt Bettinger quote, *The New York Times*, 02.04.2016.

Interior design by Richard Budd
Printed and bound in Spain by Estella Print

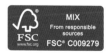

Dedicated to

Our mother and father, *our inspiration.*

Our wives, *Juanita and Denise, and **our
children** Elle, Amber, Pia and Max, for the
happiness and love you bring to our lives.*

Our 'third brother', *James Nesbitt. For
the great nights out and the many laughs.*

Saoirse Ronan. *As the Irish say, 'It
couldn't happen to a nicer person.'*

Simon Delaney. *Onwards and upwards,
me auld flower.*

Our business family. *Thank you for
growing our dream into a reality.*

Our loyal clients. *None of it would be
possible without you.*

Dennis Hopper, *for opening our first store.
You are never forgotten, our friend.*

*The memory of **Damian Corr**.*

***All the family and friends who
have gone before us.***

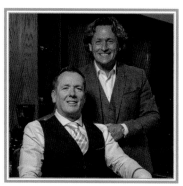

Conor McAllister and **Hugh McAllister** are co-founders of the Grafton Barber, a standout barbershop chain that gets top marks for its service and product range from a star-studded list of celebrity clients including Sir Michael Caine, Saoirse Ronan and Colin Farrell.

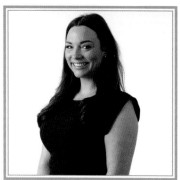

Caitlin McBride, proud resident of Dublin, is the executive style editor at Independent.ie, Ireland's biggest news site. She writes on everything from hard news to red carpet fashion, from body positivity to royal wedding hairstyles, all perfect training for this, her first book.

CONTENTS

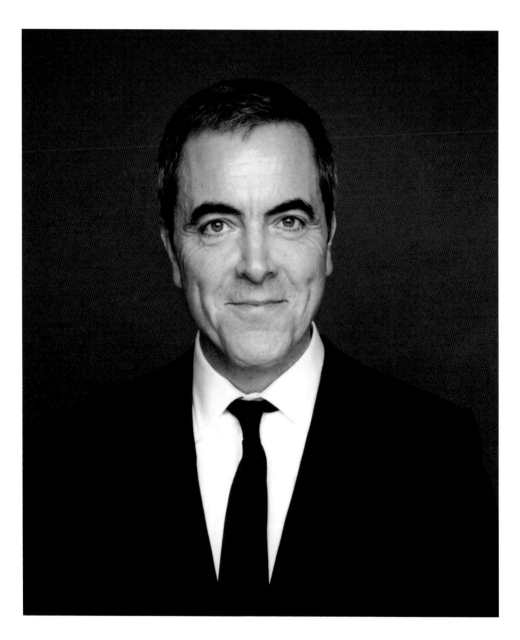

FOREWORD

James Nesbitt

I FIRST MET CONOR AND HUGH MCALLISTER when they worked as on-set hairdressers in the 1990s. Like many friendships, ours started in a pub. I had just arrived to join a film in Belfast and I met Conor at the bar of the hotel where we were staying. A very drunk man from a different crew on a different film started giving me a bit of stick and I'll always remember that Conor stood up for me on that occasion. After that, we became inseparable in Belfast for the duration of filming, and ever since.

At the time, their salon business had only just started to take off. The Grafton Barber was up and running, but it hadn't yet expanded to the behemoth it is now.

Our friendship blossomed over film sets and many, many pints across different locations around the world. My favourite memories include personal ones, like when we went to the Monaco Grand Prix for my 40th birthday and eventually ended up on a superyacht, and when we were filming *Bloody Sunday* in 2002.

That film tackled a very serious subject matter. We were doing very early mornings because we were trying to recreate those times in the early 1970s of the civil rights movement and the sleepless nights that politicians had then. One night, while in the hair and makeup truck, I noticed Conor

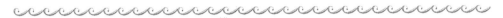

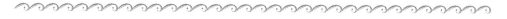

looked a little tired and he was falling asleep as he was putting different wigs on members of the cast.

I told everyone to be silent, I counted to three and we all yelled, 'Conor!' He woke up standing and must have jumped six feet!

If they are anything, Conor and Hugh are the most fabulous, sociable characters. Conor is just about the most generous person I've ever known. He's helped me a lot with charities, in my personal life and all sorts of things over the years.

They're both at the top of their game. They're fabulous, wonderful people and I've never laughed as much as I do with them.

They are generous, larger than life and incredibly successful businessmen who possess a sense of entrepreneurial acumen. Hugh and Conor never stop and they're always looking for new challenges. If I was ever in trouble, I say with my hand on my heart, the first person I would call is Conor.

As the Grafton Barbers, they're very good for the Irish economy and they've managed to marry old-fashioned barbering to the modern world. It requires a particular skill: these are boys who were raised as the sons of a barber and the craftsmanship involved in that profession is often overlooked. Here – at last! – they share all their incredible knowledge and heritage.

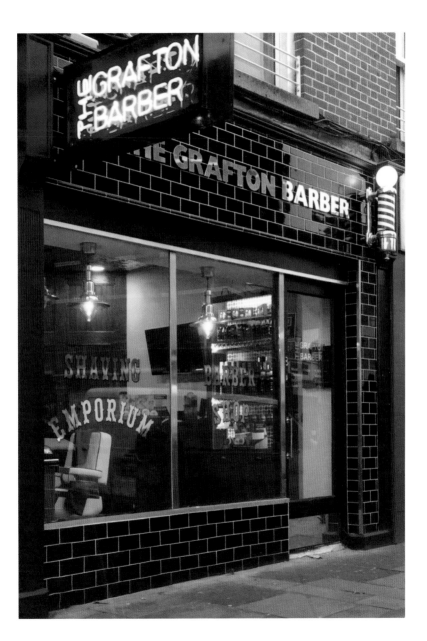

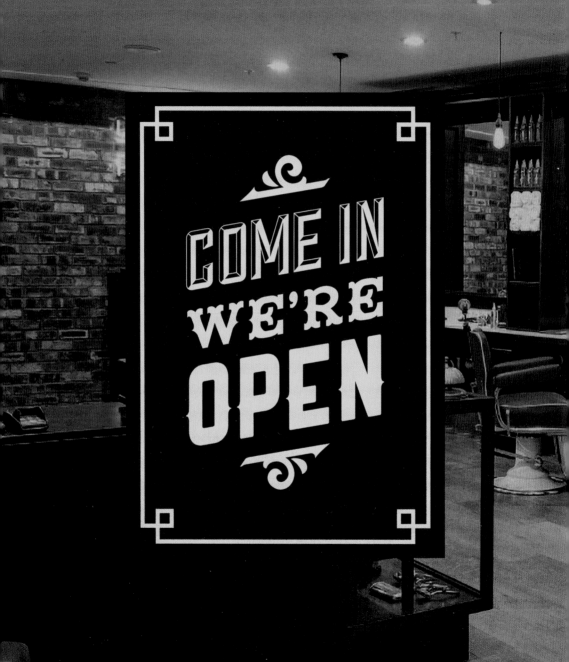

INTRODUCTION
The Grafton Barber's Philosophy

"People who say it cannot be done should not interrupt those who are doing it." — George Bernard Shaw

The Grafton Barber's Philosophy

THERE IS SOMETHING SPECIAL about a man's relationship with his barber. A barber is more than someone who cuts your hair or shaves your face; the relationship is something more intimate than that.

Barbers are someone in whom you can place your greatest trust. At first, your barber may be a stranger and yet still the only person you feel safe sharing a secret with, but over time this relationship has the potential to grow into genuine friendship.

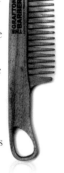

These principles are at the heart of the Grafton Barber's philosophy: you might enter one of their barbershops as a customer, but you will leave as a friend.

A short history of barbering

Since the 1800s, barbershops have become an integral part of both urban and rural communities, a safe haven to discuss the topics of the day in what would become a relaxed, welcoming masculine sanctuary.

In modern cultures, a man's approach to his appearance has evolved apace. From the classic side parting of the 1920s to the longer, relaxed locks of the 1980s that most of us would rather forget, to today's myriad styles for the 21st-century man.

Historically, barbers were considered 'barber surgeons', men who offered medical care as well as grooming. Their business premises have not only provided the setting for all-encompassing conversation, but many in the trade have left a positive mark on the world for generations.

In 1874, Joseph Rainey became the first African American member in the United States House of Representatives. In the

1500s, Ambroise Paré was a French barber surgeon who pioneered battlefield medical procedures and is regarded as one of the innovators of successful surgery. And James Arthur, a barber and civil rights activist from Birmingham, Alabama, carried an American flag during the Selma to Montgomery voting rights march in 1965 – and at every anniversary march afterwards until his death at the age of 86 in 2009.

Theirs is a unique craft passed through generations and perfected over hundreds of years. It's a role that the best barbers take seriously – with that influence comes a sense of responsibility both for themselves and that of the greater good. It's this sense of duty that is at the core of the Grafton Barber's identity – exemplifying their desire to rekindle the dignities of the past in a fast-changing world.

• • •

In 2018 Hugh and Conor McAllister, brothers and co-owners of the Grafton Barber, celebrate 24 years in business, and in that time they've taken this distinctly Irish brand and grown it from a basement barber on Dublin's Grafton Street to a franchise of more than 40 shops. So, what's the secret of their success?

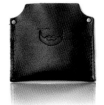

A proud heritage

Hugh and Conor are the first to recognise the vital role that heritage plays in their brand's identity. Their father, Hugh Snr, began the family business as a barber in 1960s Belfast, Northern Ireland, at the age of 15. The brothers describe him as a renaissance man who cut his teeth first as a barber, as a wig and toupee salesman, then in the car sales business before establishing five hair salons with their mother Bernie in the 1980s.

An entrepreneurial spirit is certainly in the brothers' DNA, as is a passion for grooming and styling hair in all its glory, but more than that, it's the lost, or at least dying, art of service that informs their philosophy. Service is in their blood – and theirs is a vision of service that permeates every aspect of their lives.

Such service focuses on good manners in all situations. From the moment someone walks into a Grafton Barber shop, they are greeted by an apprentice barber, who politely removes their coat and engages them in genial conversation, the terms of which the customer can dictate. From there, they are shown to their seat and cared for with diligence.

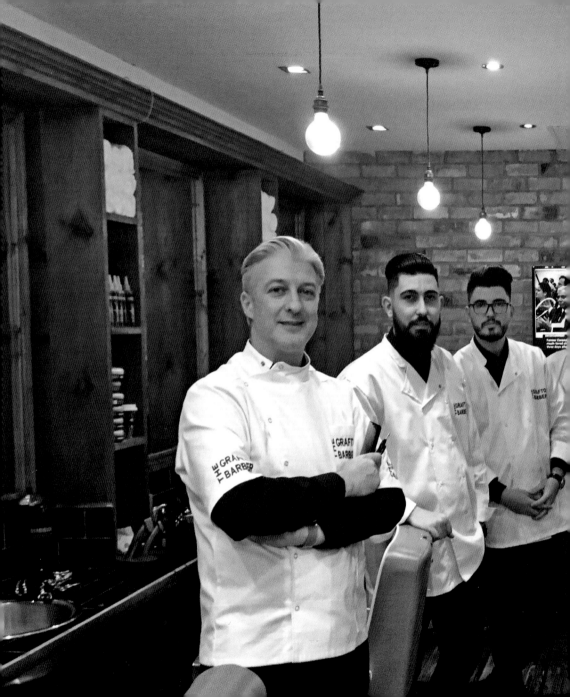

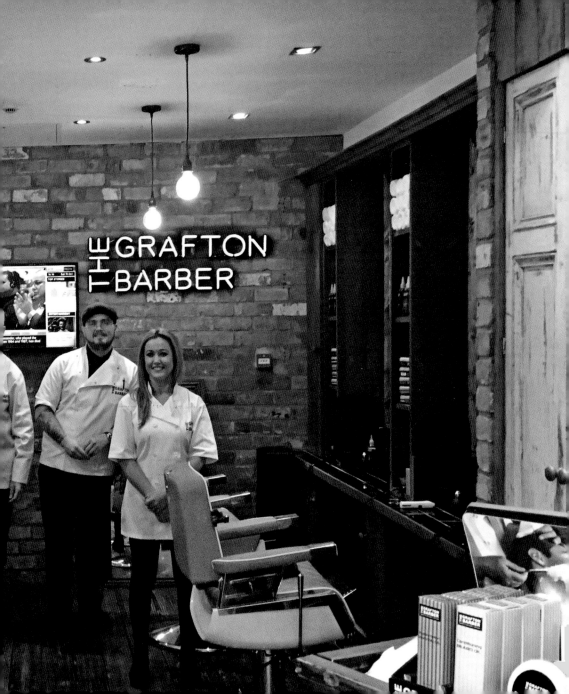

The rules of engagement

There is a Grafton Barber rule that a barber is never to ask a new client's occupation. This is so both parties can enjoy a more fluid conversation, based on common interests, which allows an organic relationship to form.

It is through these seemingly small practices that a virtuous circle of charm, confidence, decency and respect is created. Such a circle is sometimes dismissed as a custom of the past, but it's one which the Grafton Barber's philosophy is committed to extending beyond the barbershop doors.

In barbers we trust

Trust is built early on in what is an intimate situation. We all know that your appearance, while by no means the sum of your individual value, is the first thing the world sees – in a barbershop scenario you trust someone to understand what it is that makes you *you*. And so, every treatment is bespoke, tailored to the individual and their circumstances. Quality remains a cornerstone of each unique experience. Thus, trust – the basis of all meaningful personal relationships – is created.

The principles of integrity and commitment inform the McAllisters' work with each and every one of their clients. They have forged genuine, wide-ranging and long-lasting friendships with many clients, of the celebrity and non-celebrity variety.

For example, Conor began working with Oscar-nominated Irish actress Saoirse Ronan when she was 13 years old. Saoirse still uses Conor's services when on international film tours and she remains a close family friend – and godmother to his eldest child – as do her parents.

Something old, something new

Loyalty is a key factor in the McAllisters' distinctive approach to business. Eddie McEvoy – an 84-year-young barber – remains in their employ, tending to customers, some old, some new, on a daily basis. His presence creates a sense of old-world charm, pride and expertise that no one can fail to respect, appreciate and hope to emulate.

All of which can, of course, be summarised as behaving entirely in line with the original Grafton Barber ethos: be well-mannered and warm-hearted with customers, colleagues, friends and family.

INITIAL ETIQUETTE AT THE GRAFTON BARBER'S

You will always be greeted with a smile.

• • •

A door will always be opened for you.

• • •

You will be met with eye contact.

• • •

Your coat will be respectfully taken from your shoulders.

• • •

This is all done in the hope that a natural rapport can emerge.

• • •

CUTTING REMARKS

Treat people the way you want to be treated and then some. This is an ethos that Hugh and Conor's parents, both veteran hairdressers, taught their sons, and it's a heritage that has stood the Grafton Barbers in excellent stead as they serve the gentlemen – and their sons – of Dublin and beyond.

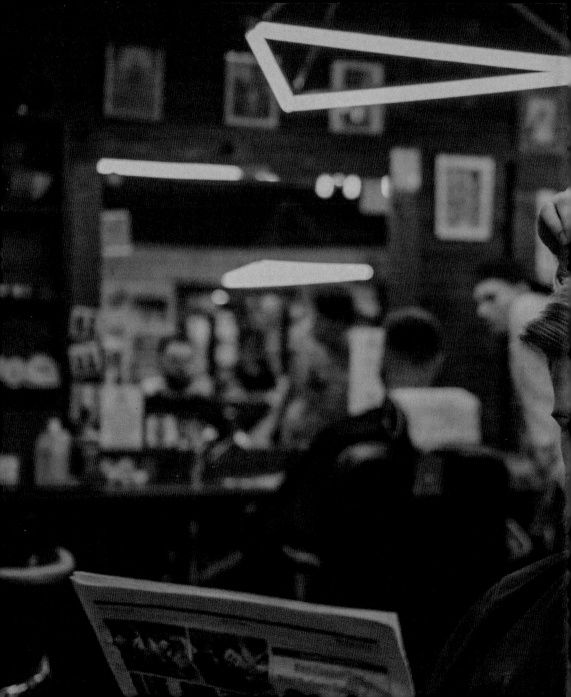

CHAPTER 1
The Art of Conversation

"How many undervalue the power of simplicity! But it is the real key to the heart." – William Wordsworth

Where It All Began

DUBLIN'S GRAFTON STREET is a thoroughfare brimming with activity, comparable to New York's Fifth Avenue and the Champs-Elysées of Paris. And it is home to the first Grafton Barber. The eponymous street is a cultural landmark for Irish citizens and visiting tourists – it remains the epicentre of activity for iconic Irish retailers like Brown Thomas and Bewley's café. It's just a stone's throw away from the five-star Shelbourne Hotel, another jewel in Dublin's crown.

Nestled amid this buzz of activity at number 51 is the basement barber where Conor and Hugh's careers as stylish entrepeneurs began.

Inside, the walls are adorned with photos of the brothers meeting politicians, celebrities, titans of industry; a pictorial introduction into the enduring friendships they build with clients from all walks of life.

It's not just the décor, with its solid oak cases and traditionally designed chairs, that offers a glimpse of nostalgia; the barbers themselves remain steadfastly concerned with putting anyone who walks through their doors at ease.

When they first opened those doors in 1994, the intention was to raise the standards expected of a visit to the barber – it isn't just about getting a haircut, it's about an experience, one which affords the opportunity to spread the word about the ethos to which they subscribe.

For example, it's clear the craftsmanship of a simple conversation is a skill in danger of becoming reduced to the practice of masters. At the Grafton Barber, such craftsmanship is a hallmark of their service, combined with the affable nature that has given the McAllisters opportunities beyond their wildest dreams.

In fact, the brothers credit their first big break to the art of engaging in relaxing conversation.

Four Grafton Barber ways to welcome: the principles of which can be used by anyone in personal or professional settings

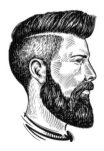 **1 NEVER UNDERESTIMATE THE POWER OF A GREETING.** *First impressions matter, which is why they remain one of the few barbershops to employ apprentice barbers – it's a way to ensure every new client feels immediately welcome. Waiting for an acknowledgement on arrival can feel like an eternity – whether it's in a barbershop, a restaurant or at a friend's house for a dinner party. Always ensure there is a friendly face there to acknowledge someone.*

2 TAKE SOMEONE'S COAT. *If you are hosting in a professional or personal capacity, this simple gesture is a sure-fire way to ensure your guest feels valued. It also offers a very brief opportunity to assess someone's mood. Did they smile back at you? If so, the door is open for some chat. If not, you know to cut the hair short and the conversation even shorter.*

3 ALWAYS BRING SOMEONE TO THEIR SEAT. *Pointing generically towards a group of chairs can be intimidating to customers, particularly if they are first timers. Conor and Hugh equate this to sending a customer into the wilderness! They emphasise taking someone to their seat as a prime opportunity to put someone at ease early on, by showing them that their time is appreciated.*

4 PERHAPS THE MOST CRUCIAL RESPONSIBILITY IS TO BE INFORMED. *Read the news every morning, paying particular attention to areas outside of your interest, so you can converse across a variety of topics. There are two questions that aren't permitted on the Grafton Barber premises and they are, 'What do you do for a living?' and, 'Are you going anywhere nice on holiday?' Familiarise yourself with enough material that you can lead a knowledge-based conversation, then if someone returns, you know exactly how to encourage them to relax.*

Hugh Snr at work in 1961 on Carlisle Circus, Antrim Road, Belfast.

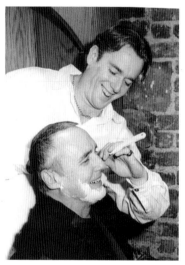

Conor shaving Dennis Hopper.

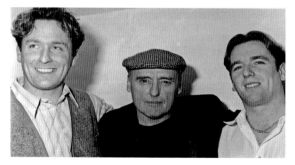

Dennis Hopper with Hugh and Conor.

With thanks to Dennis Hopper

Conor was the on-set hairstylist for the 1996 film *Space Truckers*, which was shooting at Ardmore Studios in Co. Wicklow at the time, and he and actor Dennis Hopper spent every day for six months working together. Oftentimes, in these intense, extraordinary work situations, friendships can flourish faster than normal, but still last a lifetime.

Dennis had finished filming and was asking Conor what was next. The young hairstylist explained that he was about to set up his own business with his brother. Without being asked, Dennis offered to launch it for them, a true testament to the rapport that had been built in the previous six months.

His endorsement – which would have cost millions through official channels – was free of charge and elevated their brand-new business to unexpected heights from the get-go. They received blanket coverage across national publications and radio stations and they haven't stopped since.

An unexpected visitor

Fast forward a few years and former US president Bill Clinton had just visited Dublin. A customer, clearly an army man, came into the shop, sat in the chair and put down his bag, which had a presidential seal on it. He asked, unsurprisingly, for a flat top.

The barber asked how he'd heard about the Grafton Barber and he explained that he was part of President Clinton's security detail. 'You're not going to believe this. I was with President Clinton one night and Dennis Hopper was his guest. When they were speaking about his trip to Ireland, Dennis pulled out a newspaper clipping from his wallet with a picture of him getting a shave at the Grafton Barber, and I knew that when I arrived in Ireland I wanted to come here to get a haircut,' the army man told them.

All that, from what began as just one conversation. It testifies to the ability to build connections and to the generosity of spirit that's so paramount to Conor and Hugh's success, a generosity which is repaid by employees and clients many times over.

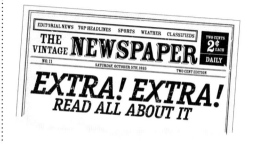

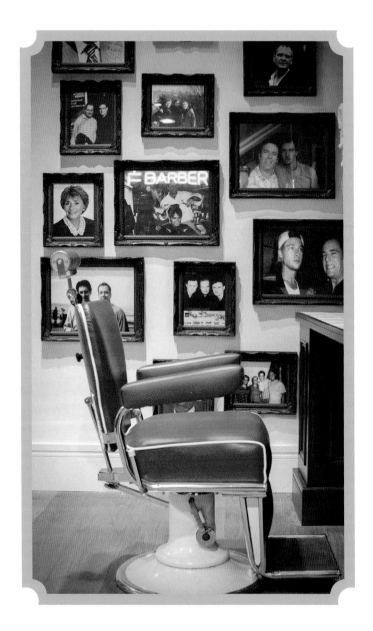

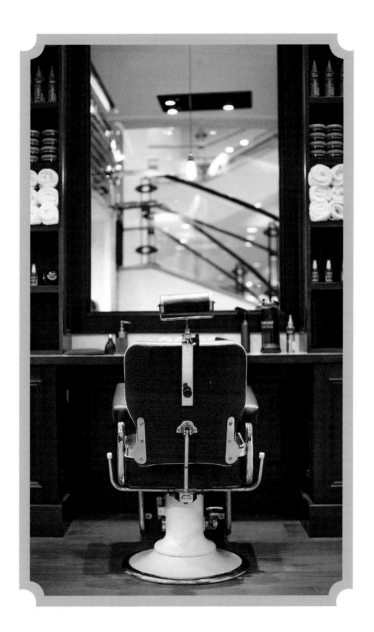

Not so careless talk

It's through these principles that you can easily create a warm and friendly environment, which doesn't just enable conversation, but also fosters would-be friendships. And, as you build on those interactions and friendships, you can bring into play these straightforward pointers to create conversations that flow with ease, humour and good grace.

1 IT'S NOT ALL ABOUT YOU. In artful conversation, less is often more. Don't ramble on with superfluous details – it's nice to tell stories in which others are the heroes too – and aim to be that rare person who listens more than they speak.

2 LISTEN. Ask questions and really listen to the answer. You can then develop the conversation in line with what the other person has said rather than simply pursuing your own opinions. Being genuinely engaged and interested in another is the hallmark of a true conversationalist.

3 DON'T BE A KNOW-IT-ALL. It's dull and off-putting. Likewise, you don't have to unthinkingly agree with everything someone else says. A civilised difference of opinion makes the world go round.

4 MAKE EYE CONTACT. This is a sure-fire winner; it creates a bond that feels sincere and trusting. But be sensible about it – don't stare or play power games.

5 RECIPROCATE. Good-natured conversation is reciprocal and flows smoothly. Mastering the art of conversation shows others that you are interested and interesting. It's an art you can always keep learning, and always keep reaping the benefits of at home, work and play.

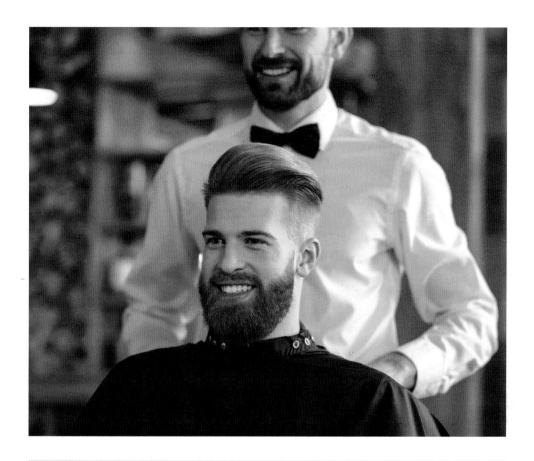

CUTTING REMARKS: The idea of treating everyone equally might sound like a worn-out phrase beloved of teachers and parents, but it really is the key to long-lasting relationships. 'Ordinary' people want to be treated like celebrities, especially when they're paying for a service, and celebrities want to be treated like 'ordinary' people. If you give the same attention to detail in conversation with anyone, from any walk of life, you are guaranteed success.

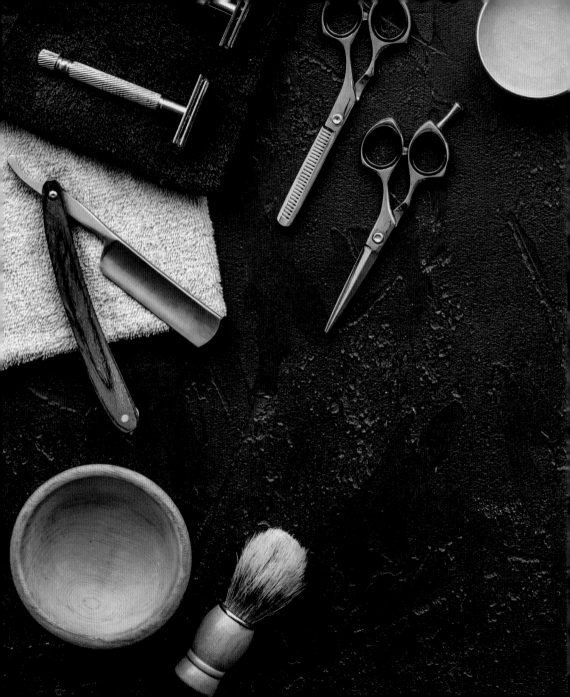

CHAPTER 2
Scrubbing Up Well

"To love oneself is the beginning of a lifelong romance." – Oscar Wilde

Essential Skincare Advice

WITH MORE THAN 25 YEARS' experience in men's grooming, Conor and Hugh have picked up more th a few tricks of the trade. As veteran hairstylists, they have seen it all – offering not only guidance and practical advice to customers, but also dignity and respect. Everyone deserves to feel their best, whatever the circumstances might be.

There is no quick fix that can beat a good skincare regime, but it can be factored into your morning and night-time routine with minimum disruption. And even better news, it doesn't have to be expensive!

Modern men are catching up with their female counterparts in terms of skincare, not only in product and treatment availability, but in educating themselves on the importance of skincare management.

Men's grooming is an evolving market, one which is flourishing, and, on the bustling floor of the barbershop, Conor and Hugh see first-hand how men are using skincare in new and different ways.

Your skin type

Before embarking on any skincare regime it's vital to first establish what kind of skin you have. The four main skin types all require a slightly different approach, so it's well worth ascertaining if you have normal, oily, dry or combination skin. You can check how to do this online – or seek advice from specialists in a large department store.

From the inside out

There are three key elements to men's skincare: hydration, moisturisers and SPF. Conor and Hugh adhere to a holistic school of thought, one which goes beyond skin deep to appreciate the underlying factors of respecting personal value through self-care.

Hydration starts from the inside out and this means drinking plenty of water – at least the two litres recommended daily, and

ESSENTIALS FOR YOUR SKINCARE REGIME

FACEWASH: Invest in two types of facewash – one for daily use and one to use as an exfoliator no more than three times a week to wash away dead skin cells.

• • •

MOISTURISER: Once you identify what type of skin you have (normal, oily, dry or combination), find a corresponding moisturiser to match and help nourish your skin and enhance your complexion. You don't need to spend a fortune on this to reap the benefits – one that costs €12 can be just as efficient as one for €40.

• • •

SPF: You should apply factor 50 every single morning even if you're not in the sun – it also protects against pollutants.

• • •

TOPICAL CREAMS FOR SENSITIVE SKIN: If you have eczema, psoriasis, acne or persistent dry skin, include all of the above in your arsenal, but visit a dermatologist and follow their advice to the letter.

the inside out. You can have the best moisturiser in the world, but if you're not drinking enough water or getting enough sleep, you won't see the benefits.

A BODY OF WATER

Always have a glass of water before bed, and within a week you'll notice the positive effects hydration has on your skin: your bags will be less puffy, the whites of your eyes will be brighter and, with any luck, you'll soon start getting compliments about your glowing complexion.

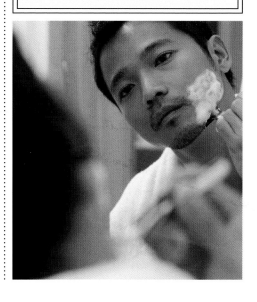

more if you're exercising. All of which is brilliant for that money-can't-buy glow that makes us feel and look so much more alive.

Products like moisturisers and cleansers are only the second step of the process and should be viewed as external enhancers, working off what you've created from

Ten skincare tips

1 ALWAYS WASH YOUR FACE. It might sound obvious, but think of everything you've done during the day – your commute, work, the gym, cooking – can you imagine not washing your hands at all during that period? Your face is exposed to the same amount of external influences, so it's important to remember that it also deserves a good scrub at the end of a hard day.

2 EXFOLIATION IS KEY. Women have enjoyed the benefits of exfoliation for years, but now men are also jumping onboard. Whether you have a beard or freshly shaved skin, exfoliation should be an essential part of your skincare regime. You should also use a quality face cloth to remove excess oil. Don't be afraid of skin cleansing machines (there are some on the market for €30) and, depending on the condition of your skin and how powerful the exfoliant is, some can be used up to three days per week.

3 SHOWER EVERY DAY (OR NIGHT). Showering gets rid of the excess oil on your body, in particular around the face, neck and back where it builds up during the day. If you're prone to breakouts, showering will help defuse the potential for new spots, which are caused by a build-up of sweat in the sebaceous glands. A warm shower will also open your pores and allow you to better reach any areas you're cleansing.

4 'GENTLE' IS ESSENTIAL. If you have sensitive skin, for example, or psoriasis, eczema or another skin condition, exfoliating can be too irritating – sometimes even water can be too much of an irritant. In this case, you should visit a dermatologist and get advice individually tailored for you. But most men should adopt a softer approach to skincare, so as not to overly irritate the skin.

5 INVESTIGATE THE QUALITY OF YOUR LOCAL WATER SUPPLY. You don't have to become a crusader for water quality, but you can manage your expectations if you educate yourself on the effects it has on your skin. For example, if your local water supply contains lime, you would deem it undrinkable; so imagine what it's doing to your hair and skin. Water softeners tend to be an expensive option for improving this, but shower filters are available at a more reasonable price at DIY stores.

6 GET TO KNOW YOUR MOISTURISERS. When it comes to moisturising, sometimes a gel is best. Every skin type is different, but gels provide more of a protective layer for your skin, which is an essential barrier especially if you're living in a city, which is more prone to pollutants. Psychologically, most of us feel that a cream goes 'deeper' into the skin, but unless you suffer from extremely dry skin, it's not imperative.

7 ALWAYS USE SPF. This one has been hammered into most of us for the last few decades, but still, nearly all of us fall guilty of not sticking to it on a daily basis. Every man, woman and child should wear SPF every day. If you think about it from an economical perspective, not only does it protect against UV rays, it also moisturises. So, if you're on a tight budget, an SPF from a skincare range can be a double act for you!

8 READ THE LABEL. It sounds obvious, but it's easy to get caught up in enticing marketing. Dating back to the early days of beauty, there were three types of creams available (all for women): hand cream, cold cream and face cream. Most of these products have been manoeuvred into different purposes to increase sales and it's important to be an informed consumer. If you look at the ingredients, and an eye cream and face cream have the same elements, then there's no need to purchase both.

9 GO NATURAL. Why does anyone need to add chemicals to a product that's intended to naturally generate moisture? The more chemically infused products you use, the more you will need, so be mindful of exactly what you're putting on your face. If you don't understand more than 50% of the ingredients, then chances are the product is more artificial than strictly necessary.

10 YOUR SKINCARE REGIME SHOULD COVER MORE THAN YOUR FACE. Investigate a body wash or gel for head-to-toe cleansing. If you have drier skin, a body wash or in-shower moisturiser can be of additional help to keep your skin feeling and looking supple.

Four things to watch out for

1 **NEVER USE SOAP TO WASH YOUR FACE.** There was a time when the only acceptable cleanse was scrubbing your face with a bar of soap and drying it with whatever towel was handy. This irritates the skin, especially if you're using a soap intended for body washes. Instead, try a foam cleanser or cleansing brush.

2 **BE CAREFUL WITH YOUR DIET.** Remember that what you put in your body shows on the outside. And, as we all know, this is 100% true of the demon drink, which is guaranteed to show up on your face not only the morning after the night before, but also with more permanent effect as the years go by.

3 **DON'T BE TOO HARSH WITH YOUR SKIN.** If you're too abrasive either with your technique or tools, it will irritate the skin and can leave you looking, and feeling, raw. After lathering your face, rub your skin gently in a circular motion using a quality face cloth. Avoid pulling the skin downwards as this can cause wrinkles – and nobody wants to speed up gravity!

4 **DON'T WASH YOUR FACE MORE THAN TWICE A DAY.** Anything more than a morning and evening routine will be too harsh on your skin.

Rugged not rough

No one wants to be a narcissistic slave to the mirror or fretful about setting foot out the door without indulging in a beauty regime more complex than that of a TOWIE star.

You can still rock the classic rugged look; the trick is not to mistake rugged for pure rough. Think Steve McQueen, not Mickey Rourke. And this is where daily skincare pays dividends – simply put, it's good form: your face is what people look at as you communicate with the world. A healthy glow lifts your mood and is an unmistakable, unbeatable sign of confidence and good grooming.

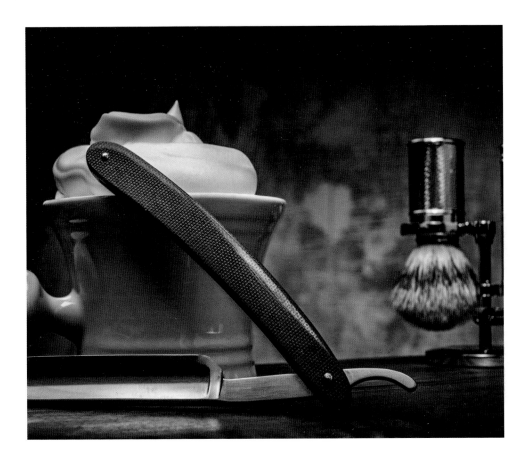

CUTTING REMARKS

Find a skincare routine that works for you – this will take time and experimentation with a number of different products. Do your research and consult the experts online, in books and in stores – and use reputable brands. Not everything has to cost a fortune to be efficient, but it requires investigation on your part.

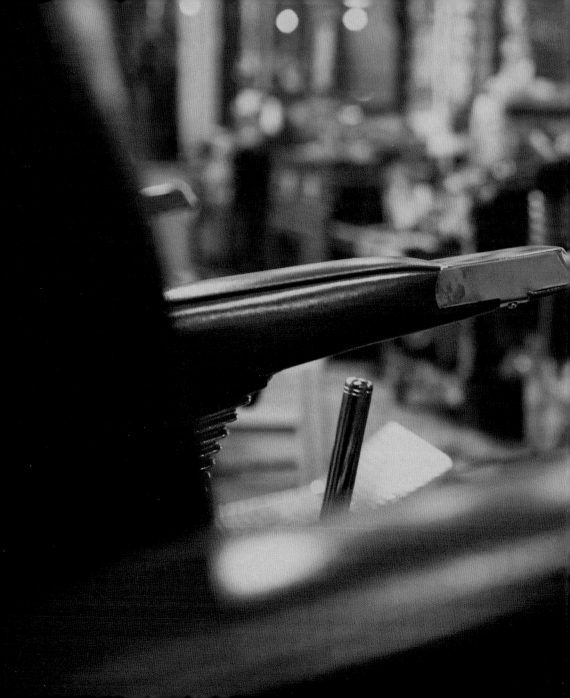

CHAPTER 3
In the Chair

"Why is it I have my best ideas while shaving?" – Albert Einstein

Shaving Dos and Don'ts

BARBERING IS A GENTLEMAN'S GAME and if there's one thing gentlemen excel at, it's putting forth a presentation of themselves for the world to see. Appearance is a matter of personal pride and shaving is a key element of that.

There is something ritualistic about shaving, a brief window of time where a man can enjoy the solitude of self-reflection: just him, a razor and a mirror. Like all masters of their craft, Conor and Hugh make a layered process look easy. In the 'Scrubbing Up Well' chapter, one notable omission was how to care for your skin after shaving, a time when it can be at its most vulnerable.

All about the beard

The evolution of facial hair trends across continents and centuries has been reported by historians and cultural observers; its impact is truly fascinating. In the 16th century, beards were seen as a symbol of masculinity and power, a belief that some men in this century also adhere to. In other instances, a splendid beard is nothing more than a fashion statement.

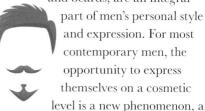

Facial hair, including moustaches and beards, are an integral part of men's personal style and expression. For most contemporary men, the opportunity to express themselves on a cosmetic level is a new phenomenon, a behaviour which is being encouraged by certain, invested industries.

Most workplaces permit a beard as long as it's neat and tidy, but in the Grafton Barber, Conor and Hugh promote being clean shaven and encourage their staff to do the same. But, if you are a pogonophile,* they won't turn you away. In fact, they will give you the tools to rival Abraham Lincoln.

First impressions matter and even if you're in the middle of growing a beard, you can still show the people in your life that you're making an effort. The 'transition beard' is a complex growth to master. It can often result in unsightly stubble or look unkempt, especially to new people you meet. You need to ensure your 'lines are clean', which means the outline point is shaven evenly. You can do this yourself, or go to a professional.

• • •

FOR WELL-GROOMED FACIAL HAIR

☞ *1. Imagine a line from the top of your sideburn to the corner of your moustache. That's your bearded plimsoll line – no hair above it under any circumstances, please.*

☞ *2. Hair on the underside of your jaw above your Adam's apple = acceptable. Hair on your neck (front or back) = unacceptable.*

☞ *3. The beard-sans-moustache is a strong look. Think carefully before you go there.*

☞ *4. Full-on sideburns even more so. If you're tempted, check Elvis circa 1969 for inspiration, not Noddy Holder circa 1979.*

*A pognophile is someone who loves or studies beards.

BEFORE YOU START: ESSENTIALS FOR THE PERFECT SHAVE

PRE-SHAVE OIL: A few drops to the skin before starting will make the process much smoother.

• • •

SHAVING CREAM: Instead of focusing on brand names and their corresponding price tags, instead look at the ingredients. Avoid products with alcohol, which dries out the skin, and instead look for glycerine and aloe vera, if possible.

• • •

RAZOR: A quality razor is key to getting started and there are more on the market now than ever before. Most good ones aren't excessively expensive, but avoid disposable ones, unless it's an emergency – not only are they harsher on your skin but they also build up bacteria.

• • •

BEARD OIL: If you have light stubble or a full beard, beard oil is the simplest way to ensure the facial hair stays healthy, as does your skin underneath.

• • •

STYPTIC PENCIL: This is a medicated stick made using ingredients from alum block and wax binder compressed into matchstick-shaped healing agents. A quick dotting on any small cuts will see immediate results, and it also acts as an anti-bacterial agent.

Goodbye to the beard?

Moisturising isn't a technique solely for your skin, but also your beard. In particular, if you decide to shave off your facial hair, most men will find the skin gets irritated afterwards because it wasn't getting enough TLC while bearded. You mightn't be thinking of shaving your beard now, but you may one day and you want that day to be as untraumatic as possible. A beard holds as much psychological sigificance as it does physical, so it's important that you remain as confident in yourself after undergoing such a drastic change.

Keeping the beard?

If you are holding on to your beard, then, argan oil, a naturally occurring plant oil produced from the kernels of Moroccan argan trees, is the best ingredient for a beard conditioner. It tackles static hair and nourishes the facial hair from the roots. The next part of beard grooming is using a combination of a beard comb and

high quality beard oil to comb it into the desired position. Moisturise the beard from the root out with your fingertips, slowly, for approximately 30 seconds. Do this twice a day and within two weeks you'll see a drastic difference – and have more confidence than ever in your au naturel facial adornment.

BREAKING THE BANK

You might have noticed the influx of high-end razors invading the market, but you needn't break the bank to get the results you want. Most pharmacies will stock all that you need for the perfect shave.

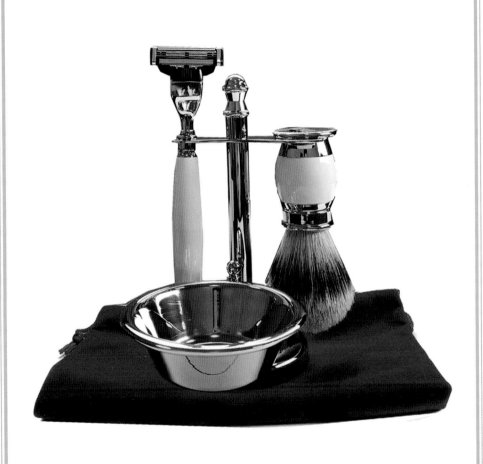

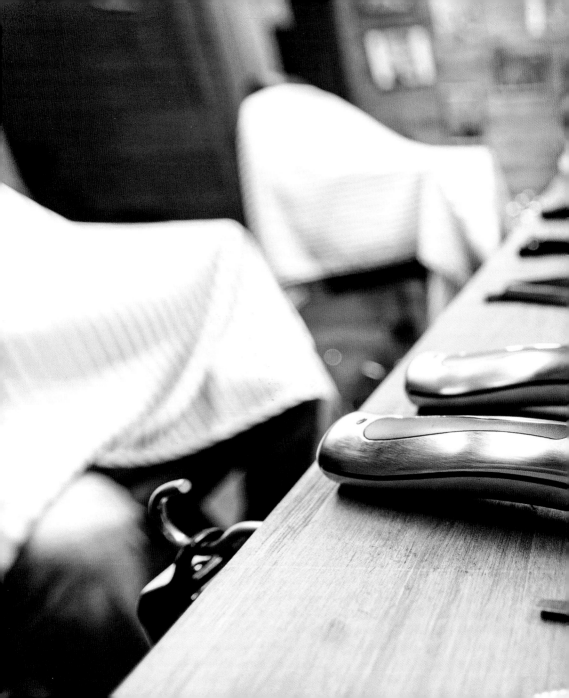

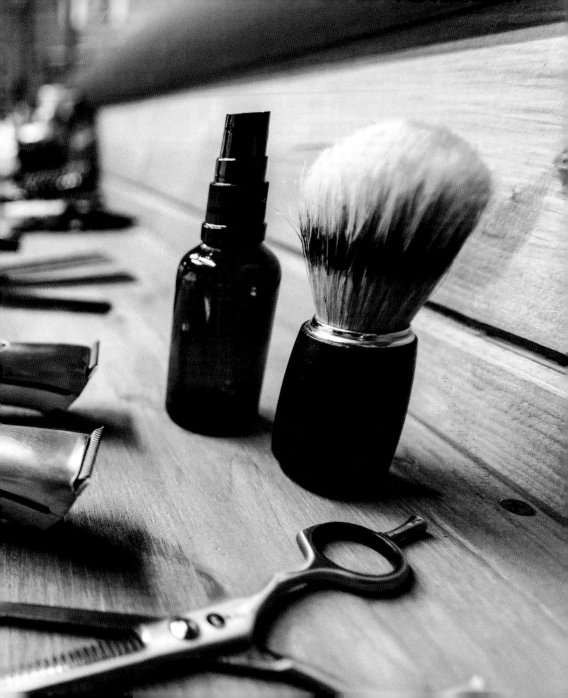

Seven steps to the perfect shave

Smooth shaving is an undoubted skill, but one which many men are left to navigate alone after teenage mornings in front of the bathroom mirror with any old razor. The Grafton Barbers encourage fathers to teach their sons the value of this daily routine. Here's to upfront chat about selecting the tools of the trade and how best to use them.

Ingredients

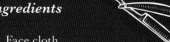

- Face cloth.
- Razor of your choosing, but make sure it isn't blunt and that it's clean. Else you're guaranteed irritation both of your skin and that of a second-rate job.
- Shaving soap.
- Shaving brush.
- Shaving oil.
- Aftershave for afterwards.

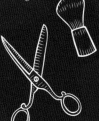

Method

1. Firstly, gather your ingredients together over a sink with a mirror. Run the tap until you get it to the right temperature (hot but not boiling). If you're not patient enough to wait for the tap, you can boil a kettle, then pour the water into a bowl and dip a towel or cloth into it. Carefully place the towel on your face and wrap yourself in it and leave it for a few minutes, which will loosen up the bristles of your facial hair while also lubricating the skin. This pause before you begin is important, but if you're in a mad dash at least wet your face with warm water. If you're in no rush at all, the steam from a hot bath makes an ideal shaving environment.

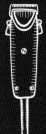

2. Apply a good shaving oil, one made with mineral oil helps loosen the bristles to ensure a smoother shave. The secret is to get the bristles to stand up nearly straight all over the face. To do this, massage a small amount of oil into your clean, warm face.

3. Apply the soap with your brush: use a circular motion, it gets the bristles to stand on edge. Brushes also provide a level of cleanliness you cannot get while using your hands.

4. Let the razor do all the work – hold it at a 45-degree angle, but remember there's no need to apply pressure or press it into your skin. Be sure to use a blade that's sharp and at room temperature. If you are someone who has moles, or you're a teenager going through puberty with acne, it's even more important to see exactly what you're doing. You can shave over any bumps in your skin, but gently. Be sure to wash the lather off as you go so the blade is kept clean. You don't need a fancy blade to do your job effectively. Like most things, it's more about technique than the price of the product.

5. Now clean your face – give it a good wash in fresh, cool water to help close your pores and seal your skin. Then clean and dry your kit and put it away until tomorrow. A gentleman always tidies up after himself – especially if he shares a bathroom with others.

6. Don't forget to check your work with care and precision – there's nothing worse than spoiling the look of a job well done with stray, neglected patches.

7. Enjoy your shaving! It's an experience that allows you to display pride in your appearance and after which you can immediately see the results of your hard work.

Experimentation is key. Hopefully, you can transform an arduous task to a few moments of comfortable solitude – with the added benefit of looking and feeling your best instantly.

Aftershave

The astringent in aftershave is essential for two reasons: closing up your pores after a shave and disinfecting anything under the skin. Shaving is something of a natural exfoliant, both with the hair removal and motion; it naturally stimulates your skin's follicles.

It's important to cleanse and then rinse with water to get rid of any excess soap. If your pores are blocked, you're more susceptible to breakouts. Cologne acts as a natural astringent because of the alcohol content.

Brocks* and brushes

The humble shaving brush – that small masterpiece of design and function – has an illustrious history of its own. Its roots can be traced back to France in the 1750s, where the badger hair shaving brush was first invented. Little has changed since those days and, although the handle can be made of gold, rare woods, ceramic, or in the past, ivory, the softness of the badger hair bristles are what determine the quality or otherwise of the shave.

That first choice of badger hair was a wise one – the bristles, being hollow, retain water and help create a deep lather – but nowadays many wet shavers prefer synthetic fibres as they dry immediately upon use and avoid harm to unsuspecting badgers. The gradated colours of a shaving brush remain in homage, though, and it's a nice sidenote that the French for shaving brush is *blaireau* – badger. The massaging effect of those bristles helps to lift the hair from the skin and the creamy lather softens it – making for a more luxurious, gentlemanly shave.

Brock being a lovely old word for badger.

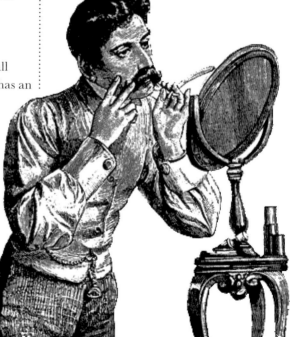

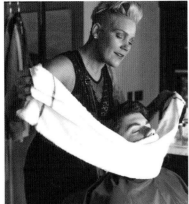

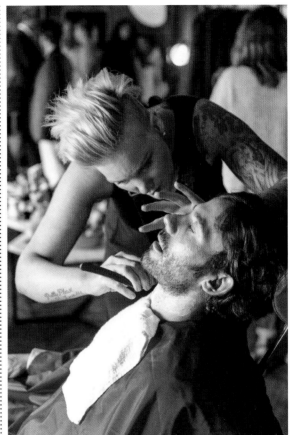

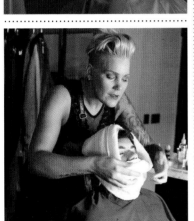

CUTTING REMARKS

Avoid alcohol consumption the night before a shave. If you were out the night before,
you're more prone to getting nicks from a razor because alcohol thins your blood.
If you need to shave (and you can fight through the hangover),
stock up on the aforementioned styptic pencils to assist.

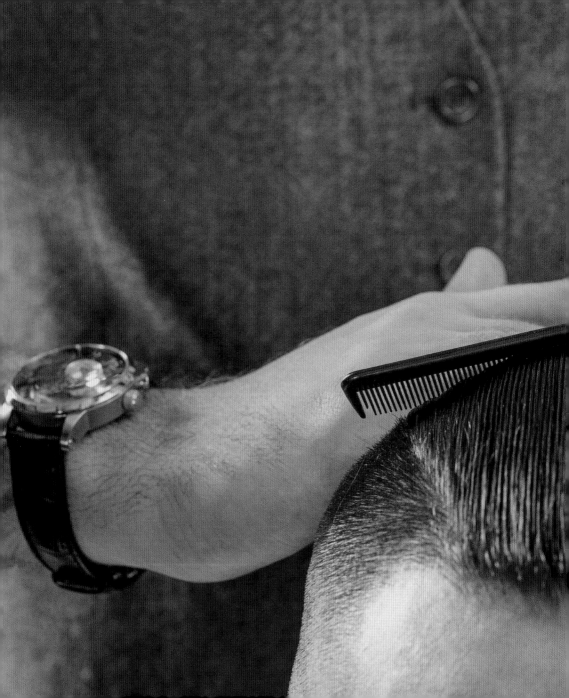

CHAPTER 4
Talking Heads

As a performer, it's really important to know that you are presenting the best version of yourself so all you have to focus on is the performance. It's more important than you think – if you can find a barber you trust, sit in the chair and take away the stress of an upcoming appearance, it's worth a million dollars to someone about to go on stage.

– Markus Feehily

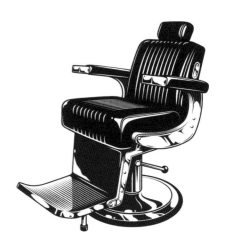

Haircare Advice for All

THE GRAFTON BARBER'S TAGLINE OF 'Barbers for gentlemen and their sons' is not only a clever motto, it's also a practical business model. When these sons grow up, they remember the positive experiences they had in the barber's chair and return once they are mature adults, allowing for a circle of trust, refinement and deference that spans generations.

The ages of man

Most barbers will cater to all age groups, from your first haircut into your twilight years, and during each visit you should be treated with the same value and respect.

TOOLS OF THE TRADE
ESSENTIALS FOR YOUR CROWNING GLORY

SHAMPOO: Good hair starts in the shower. For dry hair, try a shampoo with moisturising properties and apply conditioner four times a week to keep it hydrated, and avoid any products with sulphates (the same applies to curly hair). For oily hair, evaluate first if you need to wash your hair every day and then search for a clarifying shampoo to remove any unwanted product that may be lingering if it's too heavy for your hair.

• • •

HAIRBRUSH OR COMB: Using a brush or comb comes down to personal preference, but if you're particular about your regime, you can include a comb to put your hair into perfect position after you've brushed. Look for combs with a wooden handle, to increase blood flow from the scalp, or a metal handle, to help prevent static and create a sharp finish. When it comes to combs, it's worth spending a little extra – your hair will reap the rewards, and such a comb will have an incredibly long shelf life.

• • •

POMADE, PASTE, POWDER OR WAX: Each product serves a different purpose for different types of hair. For curly hair to look straight or for quiff hairstyles, try pomade; for thick, wavy or fine hair, a wax with beeswax will sculpt your hair into shape; for thinner hair, a powder to apply at the root will work best, but the most universal product is a paste which suits nearly every hair type.

• • •

HAIRSPRAY: Even if you want a more flexible hold, the right type of spray will help your styled hair last even longer – look out for the strength level that suits you best.

At the Grafton Barber, during a customer's first visit, attention is paid to forming a bond not only with the child, but also the parent accompanying them, who may have grown an emotional attachment to their little one's hair. After all, who can resist a baby's curls?

It's as much a sentimental moment as it is a physical experience. Conor and Hugh take particular pride in long-standing customers, whom they have watched grow up from babies into men. 'We give the same attention to a 20-year-old as a 70-year-old,' Hugh confirms, offering further insight into a brand steeped in ethics, one based on community building through simple politeness and inclusivity.

Advice on how to complement visits to the barber with care at home to ensure hair maintenance and grooming through all the ages of man.

Under 5s

The most important approach when considering a barber is finding someone who will put a child at ease. At home, children are often taught that scissors are dangerous, so they need to understand that in certain circumstances they won't get hurt – or in trouble – for being near a pair.

Grafton Barber staff use colourful gowns for children. Tiny guests are given a lollipop, or any other friendly 'bribe', to encourage them into the chair and they are told in detail about the process of hair cutting. When you're a child, the idea of something sharp coming towards your head can seem terrifying, so they encourage children to learn early there's nothing scary about the barber's scissors; in fact, it's a source of pride to get your hair cut.

On completion, children receive a diploma for their first haircut including a lock of hair laminated on to a certificate with the child's name, date and name of the stylist. This creates positive memories for young customers and is an efficient business model: by the time the next haircut arrives, parents will choose somewhere familiar and comfortable, thus ensuring the next generation of clients.

Under 10s

As fathers, Conor and Hugh know the importance of building a child's self-esteem and a sense of pride in their appearance; they have been teaching their little ones about grooming from a young age.

If your child has long hair, it needs to be maintained daily – at a less intense level

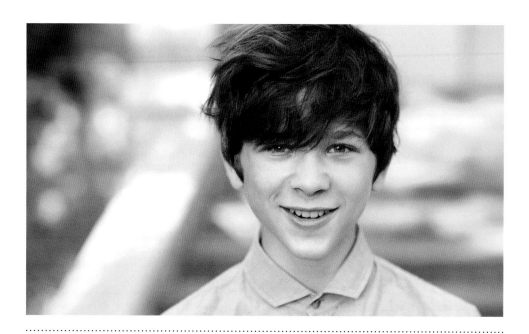

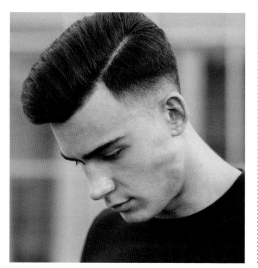

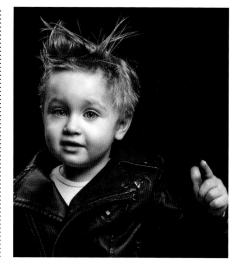

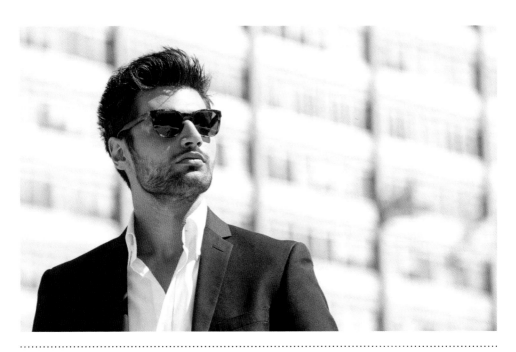

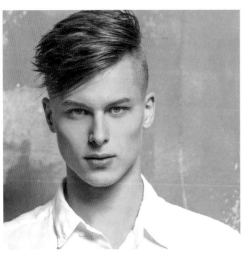

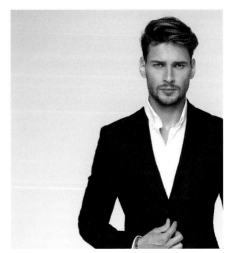

than adults of course – but it still requires a certain level of habit. Don't wash it every day, but make sure it gets moisture daily – perhaps with a gentle leave-in conditioner. Comb it every night, because longer hair, especially on an energetic child, will always be prone to knots.

ALL SET FOR THE DAY

Try to make sure that children don't get wrapped up in products and instead focus on the ritual of haircare. For example, Conor's son, at six years old, wakes up, brushes his teeth, fixes his hair and dresses himself. Such a routine gives children an essential sense of independence and sets a positive pattern for their days in those formative years.

Teenagers

A combination of puberty, self-awareness and curiosity mean the teenage years are time for experimentation and boundary pushing. It can be crushing for parents who are no longer needed to accompany their child to the barber's, but this is a marker of self-reliance for the young person.

At this stage, many secondary schools will have strict rules when it comes to students' appearance. This often means hair must be a particular length, no earrings, respectful dress and jewellery – it's an early introduction to etiquette.

When Conor and Hugh were growing up in Ireland, their icons were action hero movie stars like Marlon Brando, Al Pacino and Clint Eastwood, whose dashing, manly appearance made them global icons.

And in years gone by, an adventurous hairstyle might be a parting to a certain side or a quiff with a knowing flamboyance; whereas nowadays there's a plethora of haircare approaches and men aren't afraid to be more adventurous with their appearance. Experimentation is good, but get to know your face – a haircut that works on a friend won't look the same on you, so be realistic. Your hair colour, texture, length, the size of your forehead and height all play a part in finding the right style for your face.

The roaring 20s

After those teenage years, men are growing more self-assured. They might be university students, working full- or part-time, they might be living at home or making their mark in the world for the first time.

Most men this age tend to go for tighter haircuts because of equally tight budgets:

if you need an extra few weeks from your look, you'll get a shorter haircut to get more value, but if you can afford to visit the barber more frequently, you'll look back more fondly at yourself in pictures from this time in your early 20s.

Look at the men around you, of all ages, and see who inspires you and don't be afraid to bring in a photo. If there is something specific, be prepared to commit yourself to it in a realistic way. Ask yourself questions about the time you're willing to put in.

☞ *Will you blow-dry your hair?*

☞ *Will you cultivate a quiff?*

☞ *Will you experiment with colour?*

☞ *Will you rely on product to style your hair?*

Remember that, while you can change your clothes, you have to live with your hair 24/7. It's vital to get it right – you don't want to be matching a new bespoke outfit with a badly cut hairdo that suits neither you nor the look you're aiming to project.

The turbulent 30s

One of Hugh and Conor's pet peeves is the laissez-faire barber, who will give the

TIP BOX

Get to know your barber and listen to their expertise about what will be the best cut for your hair and your face. Spending time with your barber will leave you looking and feeling good.

• • •

And if you're happy with the results then the gentlemanly thing to do is tip the person who's worked with you to achieve that.

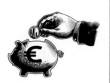

same cut every visit for 30 years because that's what the client likes. For the Grafton Barber, it's important to reinvent yourself – and your client.

In your 30s, your hair can start to go grey and your skin tone will change because you're losing the pigments in both. At this time, if your hair is changing shade, consider going lighter. If you were a dark brown at 18, don't go back to full coverage dark brown at 30. As you get older, don't be tempted to dye darker than your original

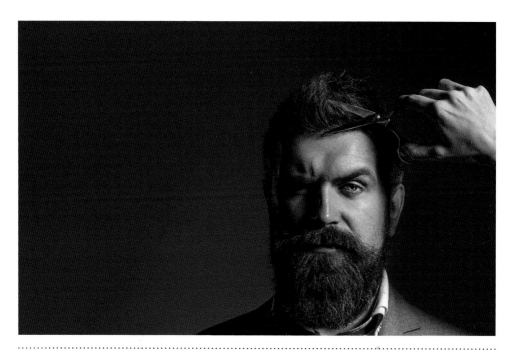

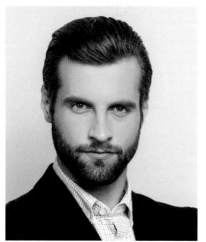

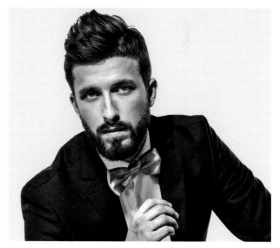

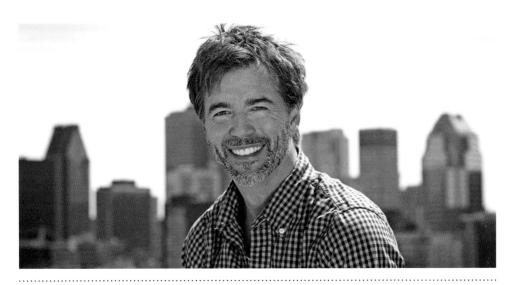

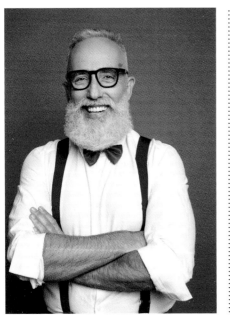

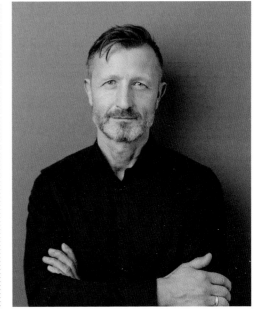

youthful colour – it won't look the same, because you as a person don't. Subtle and natural is your aim, especially if you're covering grey; a professional dye job is your friend against looking disconcertingly fake.

The flying 40s

During this decade, your hair will start to get weaker and you may begin to lose it. Hydration is an essential tool, which is as simple as using conditioner daily. Avoid a shampoo and conditioner combination: each function works against the other.

The density of your hair also changes and male pattern baldness (MPB) may have already taken effect. It's essential to keep the blood flowing whether with a scalp stimulating massage or a strategically performing shampoo. When you have MPB, it normally starts at the crown and feeds to the front and stops, then grows from the forehead upwards, which joins up and you lose down the middle.

Believe it or not, the best thing you can do for MPB is to get a good haircut. Envisage someone like British actor Jason Statham. He's a worldwide action star who is famously bald, but keeping his hair trimmed has helped cement his clean-cut, heart-throb status.

If you are going bald – don't be in denial. You'll find a quality haircut more

essential than ever. When hair is getting thin, keep it as short and neat as possible. At all costs avoid the dreaded comb-over (sorry, Bobby Charlton) and any snake-oil promises to rejuvenate your lost hair.

The fabulous 50s

Grey hair becomes more prevalent now, whether it's salt and pepper grey like George Clooney or completely grey/white. With the latter, you'll need a silver wash shampoo as grey hair has a tendency to turn yellow due to pollution, especially if you are a smoker.

A TABOO TOPIC?

When hair takes on new life in orifices like your ears and nose, invest in a nose trimmer between cuts. A good barber will address ear hair, nose hair and eyebrows. As you get older, these small touches are key. Don't be embarrassed! Barbers will cheerfully, professionally discuss these matters – however unimaginable they would have been as a subject for a chat in earlier decades.

The psychedelic 60s

During these years, you'll no longer be getting the same length of time out of your haircuts as in the past and the social aspect of a barber's visit becomes as important as the cut itself. Perhaps after years together your barber has become 'your partner in crime'. If you're approaching retirement age, an appointment is part of a fortnightly, or monthly, ritual.

You'll need your hair trimmed at least every four weeks in your 60s and it's more valuable than ever to use a quality protein shampoo with ingredients like aloe vera. Pat your hair dry instead of rubbing it with a towel or blow-drying it into place.

Don't cut your hair as short as you would have in previous years. There's a myth that if you go to a barber when you're older, you'll go bald, but it's just the opposite. It's a simple truth that anyone who has hair growing on their head will always need a haircut!

The disco 70s, 80s and beyond

The good news is that in this era you can enjoy a reduced price haircut in most reputable barbers. A trim every two to three weeks can offer the opportunity for a pleasant conversation and grooming should become more regular.

A barber should still be offering the same levels of professionalism as they did in your younger years, and most businesses should be accommodating to all ages and circumstances, providing wheelchair access and a compassionate and respectful tone among staff. Psychologically, it's beneficial to maintain a meaningful routine.

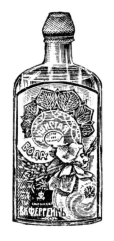
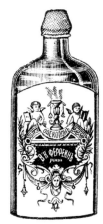

Care for your crowning glory at home

Upkeep for your hair depends on many factors, including its length.

☞ **SHORT HAIR.** *If you have short hair, you can keep it looking neat with a matt paste to add texture and control. Heavy waxes can be hard to wash out of your hair, so we'd advise steering clear.*

*☞ **MEDIUM HAIR** has its own natural flow, so there's no need to weigh it down with heavy products. A light, easy-to-apply gel can help add texture – especially if you have curls. (But not too much – the crispy-curl bouffant is best left to 1990s rock gods.)*

*☞ **LONG HAIR** is rare – except for those brave enough to venture into man-bun territory – and shouldn't need handfuls of styling products. Keep it looking fresh with lightweight leave-in conditioners and plenty of visits to the barber's. Stay away from ponytail straggle, please.*

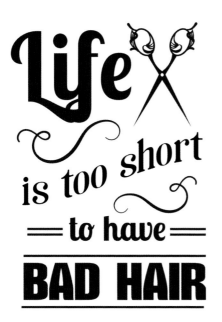

At the hair wash

There's no need to wash your hair too often as washing can deplete the body's natural nutrients. But greasy hair is abhorrent – as is sweaty, dirty hair. Showers and plentiful hot water mean that most of us don't feel clean unless our hair is clean too. All you need to wash your hair properly is a mild shampoo of decent quality – and conditioner every now and then. Massage shampoo into wet hair and then rinse until water runs clear. Simple!

A CREATIVE HAT-TRICK?

Rare is the man who gets his hairstyle spot-on throughout his life. Even David Beckham has famously tried out more than his fair share of 'unusual' styles (the noughties have a lot to answer for), and Conor and Hugh are no exception.

Even so, experimentation is a fun part of the learning process, and once you're comfortable with it, then you can always hold your head high and own it.

How to build rapport and respect with your barber

1 **COMMUNICATE.** Your barber wants you to look and feel a million dollars when you leave. After all, you're a walking advert for the business. So tell your barber what you're looking for – and the work you're prepared to put in to maintain that look. But be realistic – we're guessing you're not a film star, and your barber isn't a magician, for sure.

2 **DON'T COMMUNICATE WITH OTHERS WHILE SOMEONE'S ATTENDING TO YOUR HAIR.** A good barber will have the manners to stand back if you need to take a call, but chatting on your mobile makes their job impossible.

3 **THINK STYLE.** A barber will take your style into account when tailoring your haircut – if life usually finds you in a suit, then don't go to the barber's in shorts and a vest. (In fact, don't go anywhere other than the gym or the Dublin marathon in shorts and a vest!)

4 **DON'T LEAVE IT TOO LATE.** Once you find a barber you're happy with, then pay them a visit every five weeks or so. It helps build a real connection as well as keeping your hair in excellent nick.

5 **GOOD THINGS COME TO THOSE WHO WAIT.** In a traditional barber's it's fine to wait for your preferred barber to be free if you like only them to cut your hair. As always, you're the customer.

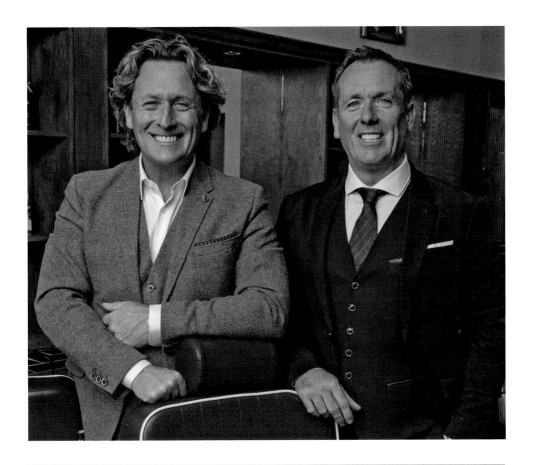

CUTTING REMARKS: Beauty always shines from the inside out. If you're investing time, money and energy into overhauling or improving your grooming routine, give yourself the best chance of success by ensuring your diet reflects your intentions. The vitamin B family is essential for healthy skin, hair and nails (it's essential for those concerned with hair loss), as are omega-3 fatty acids; but nothing beats protein and iron.

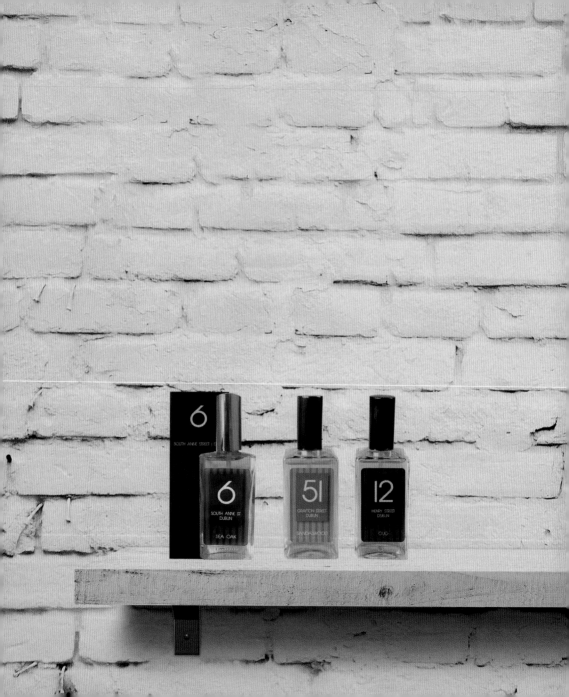

CHAPTER 5

The Sweet Smell of Success

"A man is original when he speaks the truth that has always been known to all good men." – Patrick Kavanagh

Fragrance

IT HAS BEEN PROVEN TIME AND again that smells can trigger memories in a way that the other senses don't – experiencing an aroma can bring you back to your childhood, remembering your first love or your favourite meal on a holiday. We all love the smell of fresh-cut grass – perhaps because it's so evocative of the arrival of summer's halcyon days. Scents are persuasive, enticing and characterful in ways that words are not. The easy compliment of 'You smell nice' shows how directly fragrance speaks to our senses.

For Conor and Hugh, their favourite scent is one which reminds them of the Glens of Antrim, a rugged cliff stretch in Northern Ireland where they spent much of their childhood by their father's side.

They have released three different fragrances under their Grafton Barber brand, each of which pays homage to their best-loved memories while embracing their first businesses in Dublin city centre; named 51 (the number of their first store on Grafton Street), 6 (their property on South Anne Street) and 12, their set-up in iconic department store Arnotts, in the hub of Dublin's city centre shopping district. Every bottle is made in Italy to the Grafton Barber's design and assembled at home in Ireland.

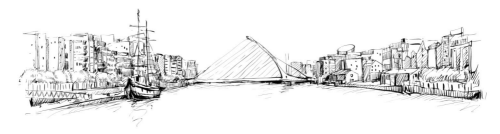

A keen sense of smell

The Egyptians invented perfume, the French perfected it and now the world benefits from their experiments. Before taking the plunge and buying a fragrance, educate yourself on the ingredients, what they mean and the best times to wear them. Think, too, about what the branding of a fragrance is saying – and what it will say about you if you choose it. Does it send a message of sophistication, adventure, sexual allure or dynamism – aside from smell it's often these signifiers that appeal.

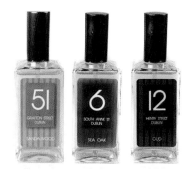

Eau de parfum is the strongest scent available, comprised of 8 to 15% pure fragrance; eau de toilette is 4 to 8% and eau de cologne is the lightest at 2 to 5%. Aftershave is more of a support to the shaving process and includes soothing post-shave ingredients like aloe vera and peppermint or eucalyptus oil.

THE INGREDIENTS THAT MAKE UP A SCENT

HEAD NOTES *catch the nose and draw someone in, with scents like lavender, lemon or lime. They are the fragrance's greeting – the freshness that you first notice about them.*

HEART NOTES *can take some time to develop out of the shadow of the head notes. They will last longer throughout the day and are usually inspired by nature, taking inspiration from grass, woods and spices. They are how your fragrance will primarily smell.*

BASE NOTES *hold more depth and remain as the heart notes evaporate, These settle on your skin and clothes, and are of musk, wood, smoke and vanilla.*

Heavenly scents

Conor's preferred scent is sandalwood, which envelops a combined smell of the sea, honeysuckle and wood. It's derived from the santalum, a genus of woody flowering plants found largely in India, Nepal and the Pacific Islands, and its unique scent has been valued by many cultures and religions for centuries, but it's mostly found in fragrances and soaps today.

Cologne is a deeply personal concept. It's something you wear, but it also shows the world how you want to be remembered. If you smell and look spotless, it shows you take yourself and those around you seriously. It can be the perfect finish to a perfect outfit – and, just as you fine tune your look and modify your accessories for different occasions, so too can you build an individual portolio of fragrances to complement your life.

Wearing fragrance with finesse

In terms of application, always spray on pulsating points – areas of the body that have a natural warmth: in the crook of your arms, your chest, as well as the wrist. If you have sensitive skin, you can massage it into

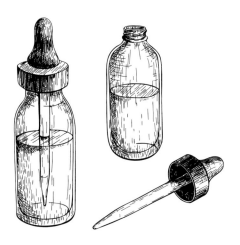

NOT ALL COLOGNES ARE CREATED EQUAL

When choosing a fragrance, there are a number of variable settings you should consider: professional, daytime, evening and seasonal. You wouldn't wear the same outfit for summer as you would in winter, would you? The same applies to colognes.

your hair, which can hold smells longer than the skin, or your clothing.

The best time to apply fragrance is after a shower when your skin is freshly warm and dry. A few squirts should be enough. You're after making a statement, but a subtle one – not that of a teenager let loose with his first can of Lynx. If you can still smell the fragrance after ten minutes, then you've judged well.

As you become familiar with your choice of cologne, it starts to smell less strongly to you. Check with a trusted other; failing that, don't be tempted to splash it on with too much exuberance. And if that trusted other wrinkles their nose at your choice of scent, then perhaps the best place for it is the bin.

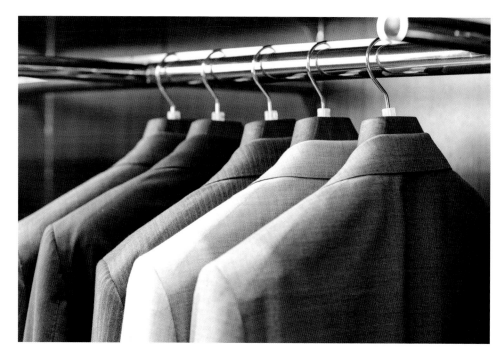

Professional

In a professional environment, you have an opportunity to showcase your personality. Perhaps it's something masculine like sandalwood which puts forward a sense of strong cleanliness that shows your serious demeanour. Sandalwood is also filled with healing properties and is recommended for anyone with dry skin conditions like psoriasis. For a more relaxed feel, consider something with orange blossom to incorporate a warm weather vibe all year round. Always be considerate in an enclosed office setting – err on the lighter side of caution; colleagues won't thank you for overpowering them with big heavy fragrances.

Daytime

Don't choose something that is too strong for the daytime, as it will dominate anyone you encounter, especially early in the morning. You'll want an energetic scent to last all day and invigorate you until the sun goes down, in which case, a product infused with citrus will send the right message.

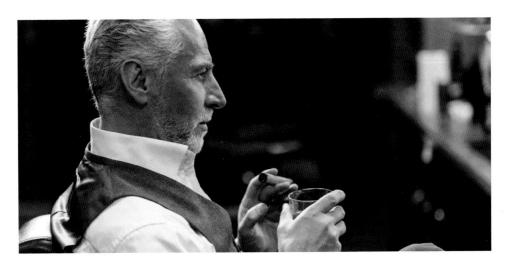

Evening

After dark, it's appropriate to wear something that packs more punch whether you're dining in a restaurant, on a date or enjoying an evening with friends. Opt for something with elements of smoke or spice. The trick to identifying these more after-dark fragrances is the bottle. Those packaged in silver bottles are targeted for the daytime, while anything in a black bottle, or 'black tie' as they're known, have been especially curated for night wear.

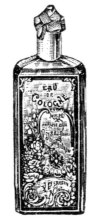

**STAYING COOL AS
A CUCUMBER**

To keep your cool in a nightclub setting, which is prone to causing extra sweat – what with the charged atmosphere, lighting and not to mention any possible dance floor activities – remember that sweating will cause your pores to open and carry the scent longer. Now is not the time to experiment with something new.

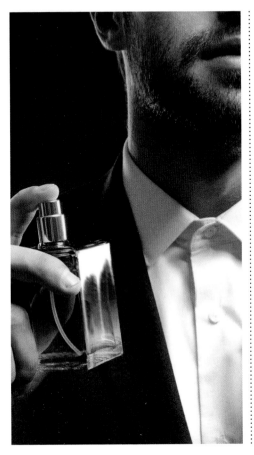

Seasonal

Lighter fragrances will match the pleasant ambience of spring and summer, so something with floral or fruity undertones will complement the warmer weather – and your more colourful wardrobe – perfectly. In winter, something spice-infused or referencing wood makes a match for those cold-weather days.

A note on storage

Make your fragrances earn their keep by storing them correctly. They don't like heat or light, which means your average bathroom isn't ideal. Best keep them in their box and in a cool, dark cupboard. Light, citrus scents last about a year; heavy and more complex fragrance can last for years.

CUTTING REMARKS

Fragrance is an invisible representation of your individuality and, as an expression of character, it allows you the opportunity to choose your signature scent. It should be an extension of you, a chance to subtly make your mark every single day – wear it as a badge of honour.

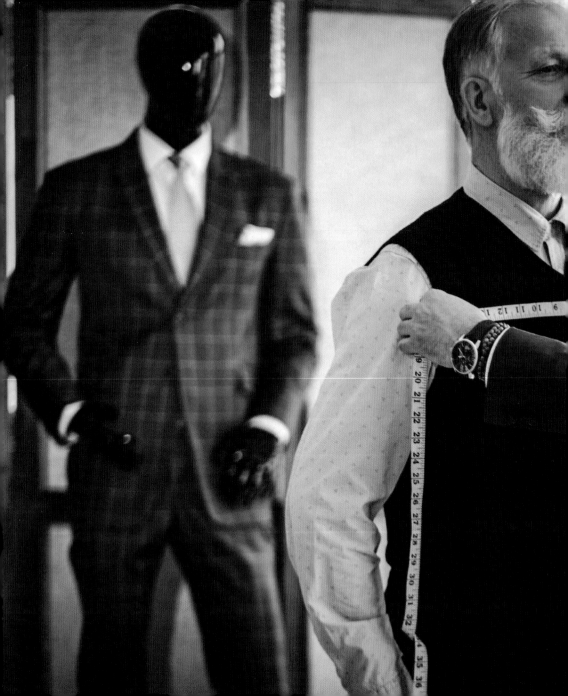

CHAPTER 6
Style Codes

"There is no honour due to fine clothes, but only to what is in the man himself who wears them." – Bram Stoker

Fashion Advice

YOUR WARDROBE IS A REFLECTION of your personality in all its colourful (or neutral) glory. Your appearance is the introduction you make to the world every day.

Dressing well is a skill, an often undervalued one, but this artistry is the reason why the fashion industry is so significant and powerful in our lives, and why a fictional character like James Bond, who first appeared in 1953, is still seen as a classic style icon.

Style is utterly individual, but sometimes it's tricky for that individuality to hit the mark. If dressing to impress feels like a chore rather than a joy then try asking yourself a few simple questions – the answers might help nail the sense of self-worth that comes with feeling well turned out. We all want an image that looks effortless, but a gentleman knows, of course, that it takes some effort.

....

☞ **WHAT'S YOUR BODY SHAPE?**
Think about men you admire who are tall or stocky, tending to plumpness or lean as a distance runner. Are there tricks you can learn from their dress codes?

....

☞ **WHAT IN MUSIC, FILM OR CULTURE** *– popular or otherwise – ticks your boxes? We don't advise becoming a Marc Jacobs, who exclusively wears shorts year round, or a persistently leather-clad Bono, but paying homage to a distinct aesthetic can be super stylish.*

☞ **WHAT ARE YOUR AMBITIONS?**
If you're dreaming big and committed to those dreams then let the world know. Dressing your best – with confidence, charisma and verve – can only help fulfil your potential.

☞ **LOOK TO THE PAST** – *can it provide that extra spark of inspiration?*

We're often told that it's what we have on the inside that counts, but unfortunately most people won't look past your external appearance before getting to know you and everything you have to offer the world. It's a paradoxical truth that by putting forward the right image, you tend to minimise the amount of time spent assessing your look.

One of the golden rules of fashion is a sense of self-awareness. It's unlikely you're headlining stadium gigs and need a wardrobe to match, nor are you a cowboy, or a footballer making €100,000 a week and looking for inventive, flashy ways to spend it. For the rest of the world, dressing appropriately doesn't have to be boring, but it should be realistic. For example:

⫸→ *Socks with sandals, a look long considered the cardinal sin of men's fashion, has made a comeback – but does that mean you should try it? Trick question: the answer is always no.*

⫸→ *Just because the sun has come out, it doesn't mean you need to leave your shirt unbuttoned to your navel.*

BEWARE THE FASHION POLICE

The fashion industry is cyclical and what goes around will always come around; even some trends which should remain dead and buried get an occasional refresh. Part of pinning down your 'look' is figuring out what you like and how to incorporate that into your wardrobe while at the same time avoiding being arrested by the fashion police, who tend to be extra vigilant these days.

Old-school style

The Grafton Barber's oldest member of staff, a man whose aesthetic is as relevant now as it was in the 1950s when he began his trade, is Eddie McEvoy, the 84-year-young barber mentioned earlier. His philosophy is a signature of the enduring principles of the business of which he has been an integral part since it was launched.

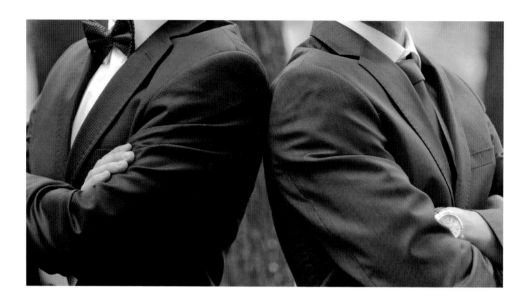

'Clothes don't make the man,' Eddie says. 'But I like to dress the best I can. I'm not a fashion guru; it's just about trying your best.'

Eddie's persistent attention to fashion and culture is admirable, a merging of the old world with the new, and he embodies what has become the 'Grafton Barber Way' – a near Old Hollywood reverence for the proper attire: from perfectly styled hair down to the right type of shoe.

Eddie owns three suits and, addressing the radical changes in menswear over the last 60 years, laments that some men 'overdo it' with their appearance. 'There's no need to show off; that's what makes some people think they're better than anyone else and that's not the case,' he says.

Be comfortable in your own shoes

Conor and Hugh, on the other hand, live by the motto that comfort is key. This doesn't necessarily translate to flip-flops in the office, it's more reflective of the importance of ensuring your clothes fit properly and being thoughtful about the image you put forward to the world.

They are both active dads, which means that when they enter their homes, they're often straight into comfortable sportswear so they can be as involved with their children as possible. If you live a more sedentary lifestyle, dressing down doesn't have to mean you're any less well dressed than your normal impeccably turned out appearance.

There is a time and a place for every ensemble. The biggest conundrums boil down to four specific occasions: weddings, workwear, casual and date night.

WEDDINGS

For a summer wedding, don't be afraid to try bright colours and seasonal fabrics like linen. If you're on a budget, a grey or navy blue suit is enough to carry you across seasons. Always opt for a neutral coloured suit, which you can wear for multiple occasions, and make a statement with accessories like a pocket square or tie. These are stylish, timeless ways to add a pop of colour and pattern. Both Conor and Hugh have a devotion to cufflinks and watches for wedding attire, to respect and honour the occasion and add a certain gentrified element to your style.

Steer clear of the gimmicky in your choices – what felt like a 'novelty' or jokey look can quickly turn to brash and tasteless. With a winter wedding, layer up for the practicality of warmth and add a new element to a previously worn suit by including a waistcoat or overcoat.

WORKWEAR

Staff at the Grafton Barber always wear black to create a sense of smartness and equality across the staff, but if you work in a business where a uniform isn't required, try a bright colour. It creates positivity in the workplace and helps foster a more upbeat and constructive atmosphere. Black is such an understated colour and you can often go unnoticed in it. So, a colourful ensemble or one with a judicious use of pattern could indicate an innovative personality and may well be the next step in courting more attention from your colleagues and your managers. If you wear a suit to work, classic grey is always a winner; a plain black suit not so much so – there's a risk you'll look like you've a funeral to attend.

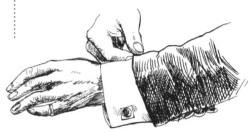

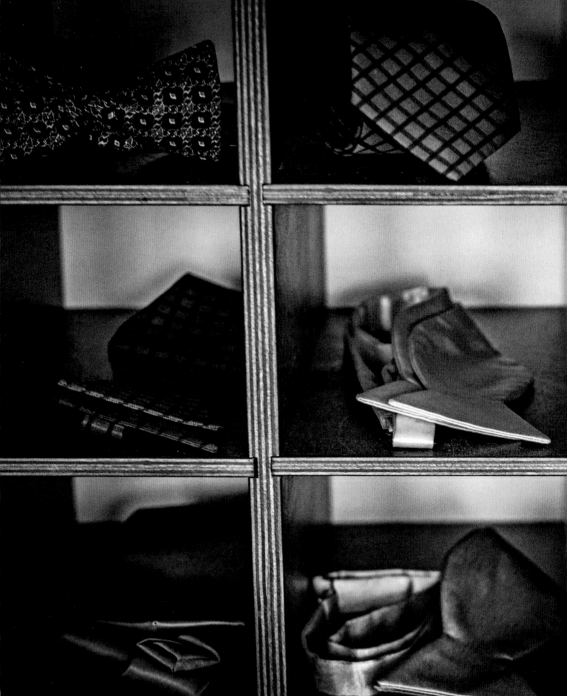

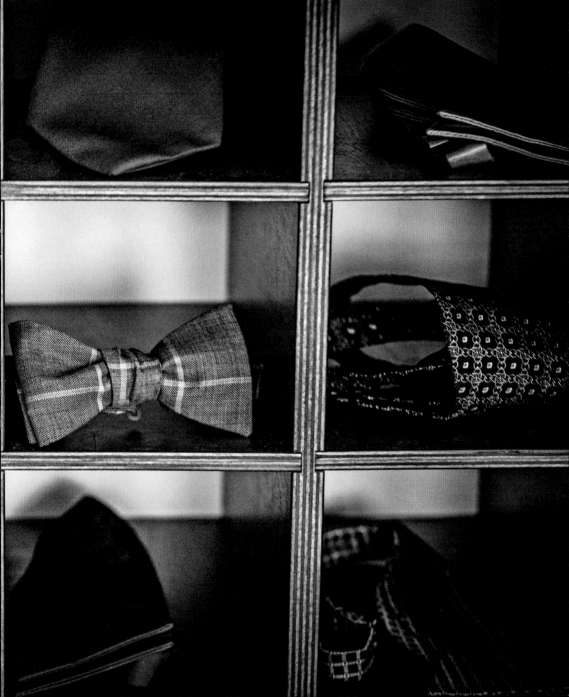

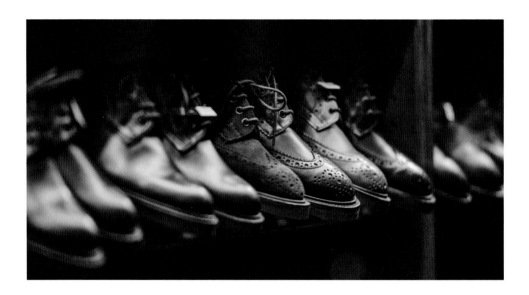

CASUAL

The cardinal rule for casualwear is dressing your age. Unlike with formalwear, younger men purchase their off-duty clothing from an older age group, so it's important you realise when that time has come for you to move on with your shopping habits – which means, no more logo T-shirts or ill-fitting jeans. Denim should be a slim, straight fit – don't chance the super-skinny or super-baggy look past the age of 20. The rise in popularity of athleisure means there are more low-key pieces of clothing you can include in your wardrobe, like a pair of sneakers with a gum sole or with a cap toe.

DATE NIGHT

The cardinal rule for any date night attire is – better to be overdressed than underdressed. It puts forward an element of respect for the occasion and you can always remove your blazer in public, but you can't exchange a pair of beat-up trainers for a classy pair of brogues.

Show your personality at its best, whatever that may be. And, at the risk of sounding like dinosaurs, don't put too much product in your hair or cologne on your chest. You want to make a worthy first impression from which you can grow if the date goes well.

FOOTWEAR: finding your sole mate

Quality footwear is an essential part of your 'grown up' wardrobe, which includes a pair of smart leather, lace-up shoes. Treat them well – shine often and give them a rest between wears. It's a long-established truth that the first thing someone looks at during an introduction is your shoes.

**BE A FOX
WITHOUT SOCKS**

Fashion is based on interpretation, but it also has some steadfast rules that will guarantee you're literally putting your best foot forward – except in the case of socks. Only ten years ago, men were aghast at the idea of not wearing socks with shoes, but now it's common practice among the younger generation. It's more acceptable to go sockless with a pair of neutral loafers and slacks, but it's a trend that requires a certain panache to pull off. Opt for easily hidden pop socks or ankle socks that blend with your shoes to avoid any irritation to your foot or unpleasant odours.

The sharp-eyed can surmise everything they need to know about someone by their footwear. Always opt for a pointed toe over a square toe. The latter, without any effort at all, will make your feet look bulky and heavy. It's a trend that first emerged as a practical one given that men's feet tend to wider and squarer, but 'practical' does not need to be a code word for 'ugly'.

When it comes to colour, gone are the days when the only 'dress-up shoe' available was a pair with double trimmed brown leather stitching. There are a plethora of options across the high street now, but three colours will carry you through the seasons: navy blue and brown for either casualwear or relaxed suits, and black for formalwear.

Loafing around

Loafers and runners are a commonplace footwear these days and, when the occasion calls for it, can instantly lift your look. Loafers should only be worn with ankle-grazing trousers, or shorts: anything longer will swallow them whole. Runners, long considered the neglected cousin of the footwear world, are now a contemporary wardrobe essential. Since athleisure gear infiltrated our day-to-day looks, innovation in comfortable footwear has been evolving, and anything with a leather sole can carry your wardrobe from day to night.

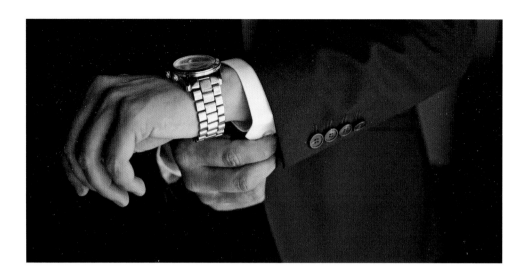

JEWELLERY: putting it all together

When done right, jewellery is an oft-underappreciated outfit enhancer. Less is always more with accessories. Heed fashion innovator Coco Chanel's advice.

*'Before you leave the house,
look in the mirror
and take one thing off.'*

• • •

Start with the simplest thing, a nice watch. Men mightn't wear a suit and tie every day, but a strong timepiece can complete an outfit with minimal effort. When shopping for a watch, consider three things: movement, occasion and size.

☞ **MOVEMENT** *refers to the mechanics behind the watch and is available in either quartz, which is an individual tick, or mechanical, which is more of a sweeping tick. The choice is all down to personal preference.*

☞ **OCCASION,** *on the other hand, is a much more obvious definition – where will you be wearing your watch? There are racing watches, with leather straps, diving watches which have all the bells and whistles beloved of scuba divers (and Rolex enthusiasts), aviation watches and hiking watches all of which would suffice for everyday use. Then there's the dress watch, whose sole function is to smarten up a dressed-up look.*

☞ **SIZE** – *ensuring you've chosen the right size is essential. The rule of thumb is to measure how proportionate the watch is in relation to your hand: if the circumference of your wrist is six to seven inches, find a watch that is 38 to 42mm wide and for wrists larger than that, try one 44 to 46mm wide.*

Off the cuff

You likely already own a pair of cufflinks, hidden away in your closet for special occasions – if you don't require them for work – and if that's the case: if it's not broken, don't fix it. One pair of solid gold or silver cufflinks can last you for years.

Good style manners

⚜ **INVEST IN A QUALITY SUIT.** *Those components are three separate pieces of clothing that can be worn individually, as well as together. Don't be afraid to get it tailored to fit you like a glove.*

⚜ **'SMART' AND 'CASUAL'** *are terms thrown around as if we are all familiar with the definition, particularly at occasions where a dress code is required and you could be faced with the dreaded 'smart casual'. But there's an easy way to distinguish between the two and it's all down to the shoes: in one word – runners. You could be wearing the finest of suits, but if you are wearing runners, you will forever remain casual.*

⚜ **THROW OUT** – *or share with others who might be glad of it – your unwanted clothing and accessories. The general rule is if you haven't worn it in over year, it should be given to the donation box. An uncluttered wardrobe is a thing of joy – and a real timesaver when getting ready or seeing what updates you might need to invest in.*

⚜ *Doing a closet* **CLEAR-OUT** *is cathartic, so once you've edited your clothing choices, make sure that they are stored and presented efficiently.*

⚜ **CORRECT STORAGE** *is a cheap and effective way to ensure you're getting bang for your buck from anything hanging in your wardrobe. Avoid wire hangers, especially for bulkier clothes, as they aren't strong enough to hold thicker materials and will cause your clothes to lose their shape. Instead, shop for wooden or felt hangers, which should never cost you more than a few euros each. If you're building up your wardrobe, pick five of your favourite items to start with, then add more over time.*

⚜ **WITH SHOES,** *try stuffing with newspaper or tissue paper to help them keep their shape. Organise them so that the ones you wear the most are at the front and easily accessible.*

⚜ *If you're* **IN A STYLE RUT,** *reverse back in time for a simpler look. Then, when the time is right, swap a preferred piece of clothing for* something out of your comfort zone and before you know it, you'll have a new look.

⚜ IDENTIFY YOUR BUDGET.

Setting realistic goals for yourself is key in trying to achieve any objective. Stick within your monthly spend until you're satisfied with your new wardrobe, which may take up to one year to curate.

Style Faux Pas – let's not go there

🖋 Never unbutton your shirt more than two down – no matter how warm it gets. The reason should be obvious. If not, I have two words for you – Simon Cowell.

🖋 If you're wearing a suit, don't match your tie to your pocket square. Instead, opt for one common colour to complement the other. A hint of blue in a tie will pop considerably more with a blue pocket square, rather than a directly matching set.

🖋 Don't follow trends unthinkingly. Take an interest in fashion, for sure, but listen to your instincts too. If you've never worn a fedora before, now probably isn't the time to try.

🖋 Avoid logo T-shirts … or T-shirts in general if you're over 25. It's a difficult line to toe, but if you must stick to T-shirts for comfort or for

taste, ensure they are crew-neck, solid colours and upmarket. This neatly sidesteps the temptation to use T-shirts to declare to the world your tastes – or the tastes a younger, hipper you might once have had – in music, politics or humour.

🖋 When shopping, focus on individual items that have a number of potential matches instead of entire outfits, which can grow stale quickly. Complete outfits tend to be trend driven and will have a shorter shelf life in your wardrobe. One straightforward way to do this is to think about colour theming your wardrobe – a considered selection of well-curated clothes of similar tones (e.g. greys or navy blues) will fit together much better than a mismatched paint box palette.

🖋 We all make mistakes and you're likely to fall a few times before finding your fashionable feet. Rome wasn't built in a day – and neither will your wardrobe be.

INSIDER TIP: Shine your shoes, whatever the occasion. You can guarantee any new person meeting you will notice. Make sure your clothes are immaculately pressed too – the iron is your friend in your quest for that well-groomed look.

And to finish – four foolproof style guide specifics

1 You might think of the **CARDIGAN** as the preserve of the old man or, worse still, Val Doonican. But these knitted delights can keep you warm when a jacket would stifle and, whether slim-fit, Nordic, buttoned up or loose they can add a certain panache that's far from grandfatherly to your wardrobe.

2 **SHORTS** are a wonder when the sun shines, but don't be caught looking like an overgrown schoolboy, off-duty rugby player or wannabe skater dude. Choose wisely, think about your footwear – and step away from cut-off denim.

3 **CASUAL SHIRTS** can be a great way to experiment with style. But make sure they flatter – slim-fit styles are more tapered, less boxy and create a gentlemanly look. Short-sleeved shirts are perfect to enjoy warm evenings; gingham or subtle florals can be a fresh change from checks or stripes, and a proper true-black shirt always cuts a dash, especially if your icon is the original man in black, Johnny Cash.

4 **OVERCOATS** – as with the suit, the overcoat is a practical garment that gives you the opportunity to showcase your gentlemanly style. Classic formal coats include the Crombie, the Chesterfield, the trench coat and the duffel. All of which will keep you snug, protect you from the weather and offer enough variations in pattern, lining and colour to bring an individual flair to your outfits. Pick a coat made from wool or cashmere for luxurious warmth and breathability. These investment pieces can last close to a lifetime; film and music icons offer invaluable style lessons in how to wear them well.

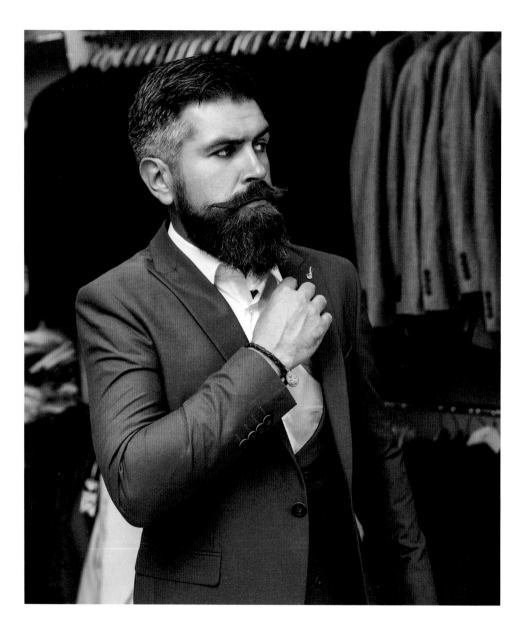

CUTTING REMARKS

If funds permit, consider going bespoke when suit shopping – meaning that the suit of your dreams begins life as a carte blanche to be filled in by your style choices. But – and the parallels with your barber are plentiful here – before you select a tailor, do your research. Be aware of their reputation, and know your own mind too. Think about the weight of cloth, the pattern, the details of the styling and what structure will suit your look, build and age. The possibilities are almost endless – and an expert tailor will be in command of the significance of these variations and advise you accordingly.

• • •

A suit that is cut and fitted to perfection is a rare, artful thing; to wear one will fill you with confidence and give you an impressive edge. Even better, like a fine wine, a bespoke suit will improve with age as it fits itself to your body.

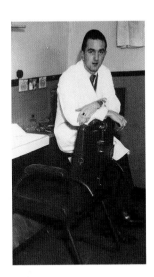

As with all things concerning your aesthetic, a man's character will always hold more influence than the jacket on his back, but experimentation is part of life – and why not enjoy some frivolity while you can? Simply put, to quote Eddie McEvoy, clothes mightn't make the man, but never underestimate the power that a pleasing outfit holds.

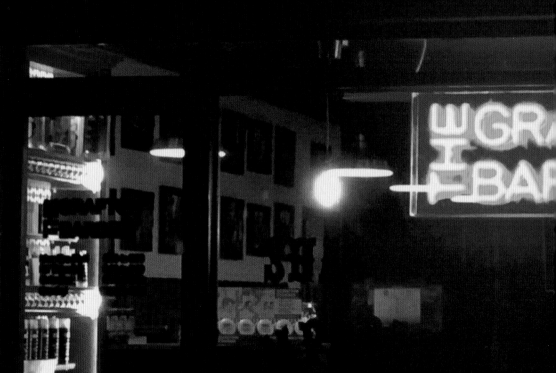

CHAPTER 7
Nine Till Five

“I am finding that success is way more time consuming than failure ever was.” – Emma Donoghue

The World of Work

'YOU'RE ONLY AS GOOD AS YOUR last hairstyle.' It's a saying that applies to most industries: for journalists, it's your last story; for doctors, your last surgery; for artists, your last piece of art. Applying a consistent set of high standards across your work isn't always easy, but it is always necessary.

Conor and Hugh pride themselves on providing a workplace based on mutual respect. They abide by the rule that they would never ask a member of staff to do anything they're not willing to do. There's an ethos of rolling your sleeves up to get the task in hand done – the expression 'no job too big or too small' comes to mind.

Teamwork is at the core of this barbering business. Franchise owners work alongside apprentice barbers – it's a scenario with no tolerance of diva-esque behaviour or pulling rank. The Grafton team is an 'army of generals' who exude the qualities that matter – attention to detail, punctuality, good grace and knockout barbering skills. Those who excel are promoted through the ranks. There is a commitment that staff will be trained to the highest level and be given the opportunity

---

OPERATING SYSTEMS

In an increasingly digital economy dominated by emerging technologies and relentless company restructuring, human interaction can feel like a luxury of days gone by. The Grafton Barber is a self-styled 'old school' operation which prides the classic principles of service above all else. Surely a factor in long-lasting success and an even longer list of return clients?

to progress. In fact, at present, all 42 franchise owners are previous employees with extensive, hands-on barbershop experience.

In pole position

In the early 19th century, barbers doubled as 'barber surgeons', where they might multi-task a haircut alongside a bloodletting. Those traditional red and white stripes on a barber's pole are rumoured to be an indicator of bandages and blood . . .

Historically, around Europe and the United States, barbers enjoyed a position as a pillar of the community, both in their necessary function of cutting hair and hosting a convivial atmosphere for men to socialise. These principles still stand – though bloodletting has fallen by the wayside, thank goodness.

Now, in the 21st century, Conor and Hugh vow to bring that same influence to each locale with courteous business practices. These include treating staff with dignity and respect, while incorporating contemporary advantages into their 'old school' requirements to create a purposeful freshness and energy that drives all aspects of the business.

Their workplace rules are formal, but realistic – and have application in many working environments.

☞ *Staff must wear all black – and no sneakers.*

☞ *Clothes should be ironed head to toe.*

☞ *It goes without saying that everyone must make sure their hair is tidy and their body smells fresh with deodorant and cologne.*

Regardless of profession, it's rare for anyone now to stay in the same company for 40 years as past generations did – studies show that millennials expect to stay a maximum of three years in a job before moving – and the job market is increasingly competitive.

Across all age groups and industries, upskilling is a requirement for progression. If you're seeking career success, then research and action the following.

☞ *What training opportunities, if any, are available through your workplace?*

☞ *Are there any courses you can study to boost your CV, whether they are weekend brush-ups or in-depth, part-time degrees?*

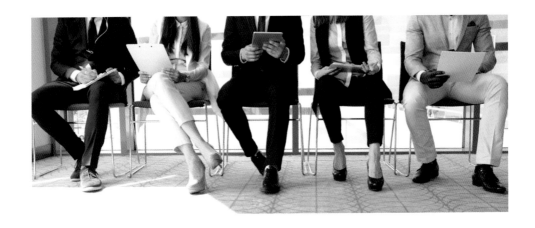

Rising to the top

In most businesses, your skill level is only 50% of the job – if you don't have a matching personality, you might find yourself becoming professionally stagnant.

If socialising doesn't come naturally to you, take a look at what your colleagues are up to and be flexible – listen and learn, engage with the workplace in a way that makes a positive, vital contribution and brings a sense of energy and respect to the business. It never does any harm to fake that feeling of connection until you make it – and it becomes sincerely felt.

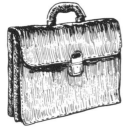

THREE TIPS FOR TROUBLE-FREE WORKPLACE RELATIONS

1 *Show genuine interest in the lives of others – but be aware of propriety and don't overstep boundaries.*

2 *Humour helps life run more smoothly – but don't be the office joker and stay away from anything even remotely 'off-colour'.*

3 *Be respectful of others' workloads. Don't be that colleague known for constantly distracting, prevaricating and getting in the way.*

Some people work to live and others live to work. If you're lucky, your workplace is not only a haven for you professionally, but an opportunity for you to make friends, meet new people and learn at every opportunity. This kind of culture is one the McAllisters work tirelessly to foster, with the result that they have left their imprint as two of Ireland's most dynamic entrepeneurs.

Nice work!

You may spend more time at the office than you do at home – an all too familiar trope for 21st-century workers, so use that opportunity to not only further yourself professionally, but personally too. Genuine friendships can be formed (some of which will outlast your terms of employment if you're lucky), and both your personal and professional skills are transferable to these different aspects of your life. If you're known in the workplace for your work ethic and affability, then why not incorporate some of those traits at home too? Likewise, you might be a hit in your house and famous for keeping a cool head or knowing the right time to break the ice with a joke.

Coffee and doughnuts make the world go round. Why not treat your colleagues to a Twin Peaks inspired Friday morning pick-me-up?

STOCKTAKE

Take stock of your valuable traits and ask your loved ones for any characteristic they appreciate most about you – it might be the secret weapon you never knew you had in your workplace arsenal.

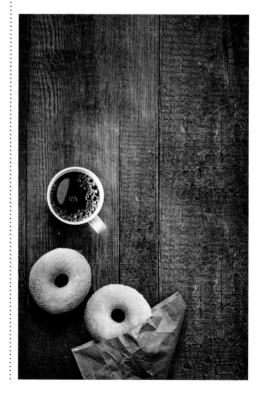

First impressions matter

And few first impressions matter more than a job interview. Here are a dozen pointers to ensure your initial introductions create the right impact.

1 BE PUNCTUAL. There is no room for flexibility on this. It is not only your own time that should be valued, but also that of your interviewer. Remember the old adage that if you're on time, you're late. This is especially true of an interview.

2 DRESS APPROPRIATELY. Research the dress code for the environment you'll potentially be working in and mimic that. If you're applying for a job in retail, you might not be required to wear a suit, but in most offices, a shirt and tie is required. Think about what your accessories say about you – a pen can be a real style statement (the chewed-on biro excepted), as can your bag (messenger or briefcase?). It's always better to be overdressed, especially for the first meeting, as it is for a date. As people practised in either of these fields will tell you, the similarities between a date and an interview are frighteningly plentiful.

3 SHAKE HANDS. The psychology behind a firm handshake might be as outdated as drinking gin at lunchtime, but its impact remains the same. Be sure to shake someone's hand as a mark of respect and gratitude for their time. When you make physical, courteous contact, it automatically breaks down barriers and puts you at ease.

4 A CONFIDENT DEMEANOUR has a great deal of impact; it bolsters your sense of self and conveys sincerity and authority. Sit up straight, maintain eye contact – and don't fiddle, fidget, slouch or hunch. Crossing your arms can be interpreted as aggressive – avoid it, unless you're a wannabe door supervisor.

5 LET THE PERSON INTERVIEWING YOU SIT DOWN FIRST. This is their domain and they are calling the shots. By allowing them that, it shows you are aware of the power dynamic. Similarly, allow the interviewer to wrap up the conversation. They are in control and it's their time you are being included in. Read their signals carefully and be willing to accept the end of the exchange at that point.

6 COME PREPARED. Print out at least three copies of your CV – one, or two, for the interviewers, and one for yourself as a reference sheet. If you work in an industry where printouts or a digital demonstration is possible, ensure all technologies are compatible and you've completed at least two test runs in advance. Don't faff about with these kinds of details – it comes across as deeply unprofessional and fast becomes that toxic combination of stressful and dull for everyone involved.

7 BE HONEST. Don't be afraid of articulating everything you've achieved up to this date and share your accomplishments. If you worked in a different industry previously, then highlight earlier accomplishments that are applicable to any industry, like teamwork, leadership and commitment. Some employers exclusively hire 'Yes Men', but you need to evaluate if that's the correct environment for you. Most employers will appreciate your authenticity, but will offer in-house training programmes to allow speedy upskilling.

8 MAKE SURE YOUR MOBILE PHONE IS OFF – in fact, make sure it's out of sight too. Even the buzzing of a mobile phone on vibrate can be enough to perturb your interviewer, while simultaneously showing a lack of attention to detail and lack of esteem for their time. Never ever answer a phone in an interview. (Ditto for that first date.)

9 USE YOUR WORDS WISELY. While remembering all of the above, relax as much as possible. If there is camaraderie building, enjoy that, but remember that this is still a professional setting. You are both there to do a job and over-familiar colloquialisms like, 'pal', 'bud' or 'dude' are not welcome in your interview vocabulary.

10 ASK QUESTIONS. If you have particular curiosities or concerns, now is the time to ask, whether it's related to workflow, hours, resources and programmes you might be using – this is as much your time as it is the interviewer's and you are potentially a valuable asset. Never ask about salary in the first round of interviews – if you receive a call for a follow-up interview or a notification you've received the job, then a salary negotiation (if applicable) can begin.

11 BE YOURSELF. If you're a gregarious character, then let that shine – it might be just what they're looking for. Be conversational, enthusiastic and honest – but don't flirt and don't name drop either. It's unprofessional and far too 'try hard'. If you're more reserved, there's nothing wrong with that. Show your flexibility and willingness to learn new things or 'how it's done' in a new workplace. You don't know the personality traits they're hoping will assimilate best with an existing team, only what you bring to the table and that is your USP.

12 POST INTERVIEW, don't throw away your good work if the outcome's disappointing. Be gracious, well-mannered and don't burn bridges – a job interview fail often yields unexpected wins.

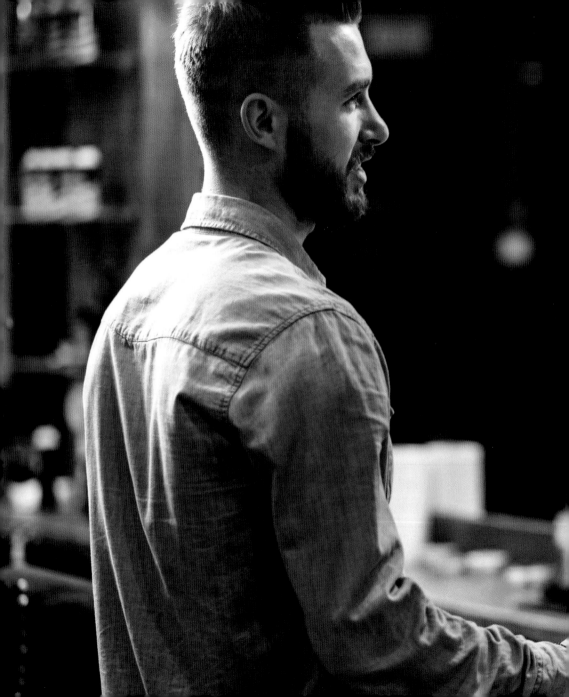

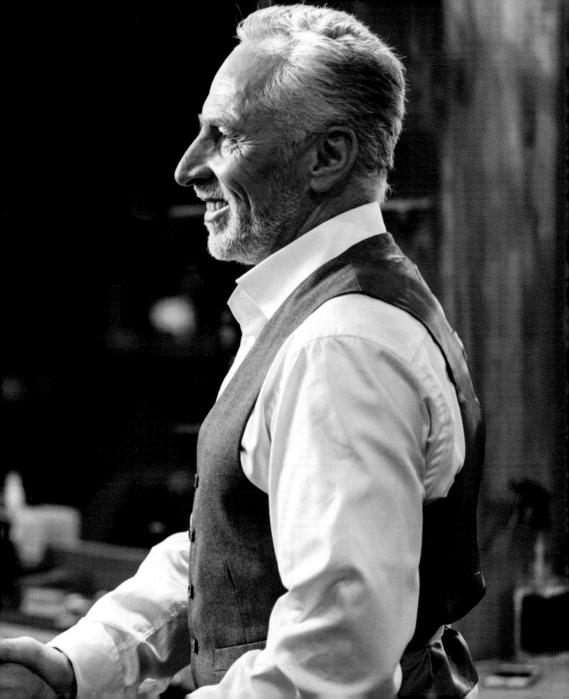

Workplace protocol: the unspoken codes

When you've landed the job of your dreams – or the job you hope might become a dream – be a paragon of workplace civility. Lead from the front with these rules that transform a work environment into a palace of politesse and respect.

1 Those who **ENJOY MEETINGS** are few and far between. So, always be prepared, punctual and keep to the point. Making a meeting purposeful really is that easy – and afterwards everyone can get on with their work.

2 For many of us, that work involves **ENDLESS EMAILS.** Again, be prompt and purposeful in your replies. It's always better to err towards the formal rather than the inappropriate, sarcastic or slapdash. When in doubt, pick up the phone or arrange a face-to-face conversation – you'll be surprised at how effective it can be.

3 **MIND YOUR BOUNDARIES.** Don't get entangled in politics, disrespecting others or office 'romances'. These things rarely end well. Make sure your 'water cooler' chat is sociable, upbeat and genuine. And keep your conduct courteous – you're there to work, not hang out. Don't trash talk or badmouth anyone from the lowest to the highest, whether inside or outside the organisation.

4 The **TEAM PLAYER** is a cliché, true, but they have qualities we all admire and love to emulate. Among these are the steadfast ability to keep emotions in check – whether it's stress, anger or troubles of the heart – and a refusal to get caught up in the inevitable unpleasantness of a 'blame culture'. A team player is always willing to put their hand up if something goes wrong rather than point the finger of blame at another.

5 If you're **THE BOSS** then take your responsibilities seriously – don't patronise your staff, but seek to keep morale high by offering clear procedures, a relaxed and productive atmosphere, a listening ear and an understanding of how other people's skillsets and attitudes fit together. Recognise your staff's strengths and praise them promptly for work done well. Don't neglect to develop your own aptitudes, and set an example you can be proud of.

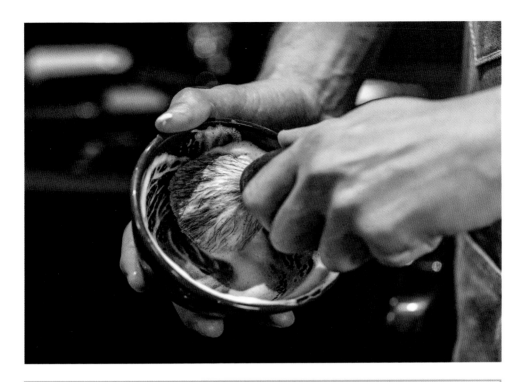

CUTTING REMARKS

It's a simple truth that the modern workplace must be one of character and challenge to appeal to the best talent. Employees bring high expectations and hopes to work: they seek out places where their passions and skills can build meaningful success with other ambitious, focused folk. But it's not always so simple to create somewhere for excellence to flourish.

• • •

Whatever your level of responsibility for workplace culture, you'll find that fairness, motivation, transparency, flexibility and trust – along with those good-hearted perks that show genuine care – go a long way towards enabling growth for a business and its individuals.

Passenger
Mr. Last Name
Destination
Dubai
Departing
0:45
Seat
A1

CHAPTER 8

Broadening Horizons

"Your feet will take you where your heart is." – Irish proverb

Travelling Hopefully

WHETHER YOU'RE PLANNING A city break, a round-the-world trip or a lengthy holiday, your attitude to packing should remain the same: bring practical pieces interspersed with some joyful bits of frivolity – because you're on your holiday, after all. Garment bags and multiple pairs of sunglasses may seem excessive, but if you cherish quality over quantity, they can be more functional in creating the perfect outfit than multiple pairs of shorts or trousers.

Packing requires a near-professional skill level in order to select the perfect items of apparel, how to wear them, and ways to put your best foot forward once it touches the ground in your new destination.

Before you embark on the packing process you'll need to select the correct luggage – a leather hold-all for a weekend away or a suitcase on wheels for a longer break? Forward planning is essential and, fortunately, Conor and Hugh have decades of experience at making the most of international travel.

Jet setter

Conor has been lucky enough to enjoy five-star trips around the world travelling with Irish actress Saoirse Ronan, since her first Oscar nomination at the age of 13. Since being welcomed by Saoirse and her parents into the inner circle of one of Hollywood's brightest talents, Conor has been blessed with plenty of international VIP travel, including private jets and boundless five-star hotels. (Not to mention the invaluable opportunity to prank call superstar actors like Ed Harris!)

The glam squad

On international press tours for movies, 'the talent' are flown to a number of key cities to promote their newly released film. On these trips they attend dozens of red carpet events and participate in hundreds of interviews over the course of a fortnight.

All eyes might be on the film's star, but for the 'glam squad', including hairstylists and makeup artists, there is huge pressure to not only act, but look professional; the fundamental aspects of which apply to anyone travelling on business in any industry. Try these tips to work a glamorous jet-set mystique.

Don't wear a tracksuit or shorts on the plane – you'll look slack not chilled. Dress properly in the public areas of your hotel too.

Be polite to everyone – starting with cabin crew. Continue with the charm and formality at your hotel – and tip staff as appropriate.

If non-stop proximity to professional colleagues starts to feel claustrophobic, play the exercise card. A half-hour gym session or run will leave you feeling refreshed and give everyone a break from each other.

When you're dining out, take the opportunity to enjoy a cuisine that's perhaps not as familiar to you as your own. It's good to eat like a local rather than a tourist, but be gracious and remember your manners. If you're uncertain what to try, take your lead from others.

Getting on board

The less alluring side of the jet-set lifestyle is the reality of packing everything needed for a high maintenance six-week trip into one suitcase.

While on *The Lovely Bones* promotional tour, hosted by Paramount Pictures in 2009, Conor traversed Europe, Asia and the United States with a single 22-kilo suitcase. That's one way to focus your mind on what's needed and what isn't. Here he shares insider advice on how to pack for a whirlwind trip, whether you're staying at the The Ritz Carlton or flying with a budget airline and spending your nights in an ordinary business hotel.

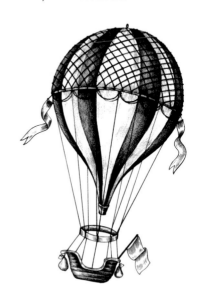

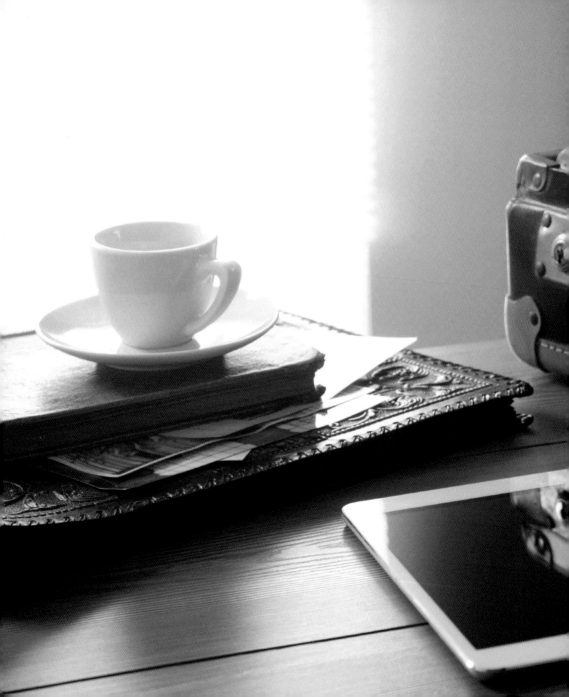

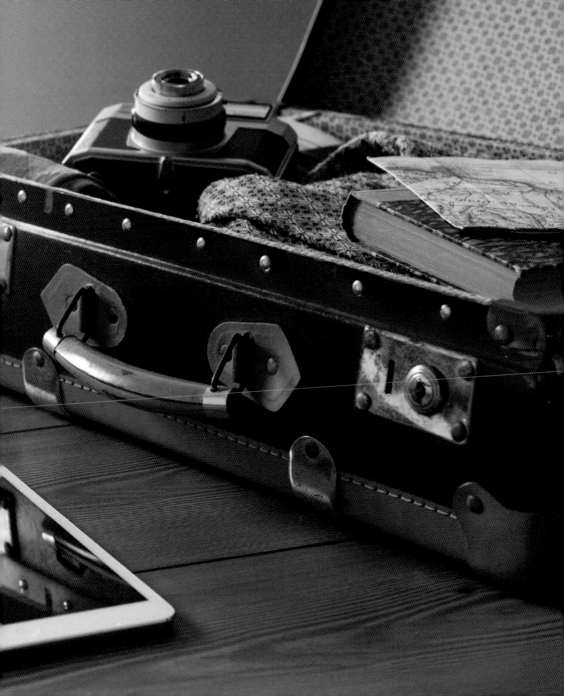

Ten ways to become a packing whizz

1 Pack three different pairs of trousers. There is little need to pack more than that as most hotels and residences have laundry services available. It's a prime way to save space.

2 Bring a shirt for each day of your trip. If it's longer than one week, you can have them laundered before your next seven days.

3 Don't pack a jacket. Wear it on the plane as an easy space saver!

4 Pack your shaving tools selectively. For a short trip, 100ml of shaving oil and a shaving brush should suffice. You can buy razor blades on arrival.

5 If you need to bring electrical equipment, it's often more practical to buy voltage converters on arrival, as they are unnecessarily bulky. Remember any chargers and so on that you might need for your tech.

6 Bring a moisturiser in your carry-on case. Top up your skin during the flight, especially if it's long-haul. Regularly hydrating your skin prevents the plane's air-conditioning system drying it out too much.

7 A sample size bottle of cologne will instantly freshen you up at the end of a long-haul flight.

8 Stay away from alcohol on a plane. The air on a plane tends to be really dry and you will find yourself dehydrating much faster than at ground level – which will show on your skin as well as your mood. Stick to sparkling water; you'll feel a million times better.

9 Don't forget to take a book if that's your thing – it'll stave off travel ennui and a carefully chosen tome can offer the perfect insight into the history and culture of your new destination. Or even just a great read!

10 Ditto your gym kit. Even if your hotel doesn't offer a super-luxe spa experience, or your getaway destination isn't the perfect tropical island, a swim or a run in a different environment is an exhilarating way to get a feel for a place. Check out the local pool or go for a run that takes in the sights of an unknown city.

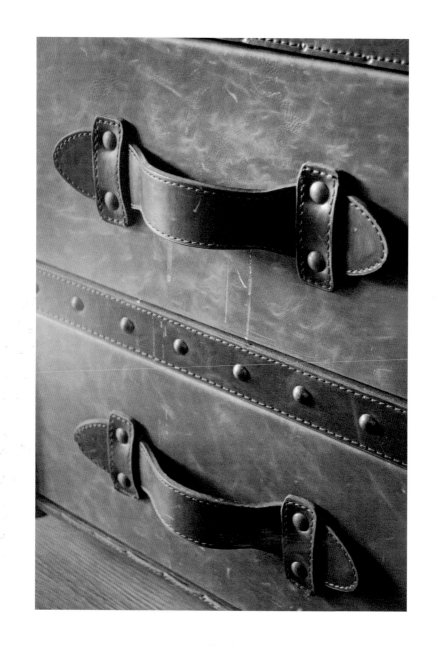

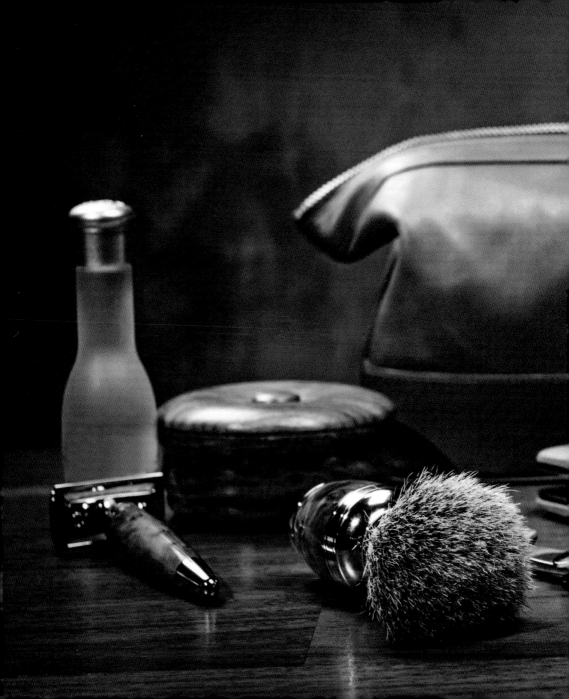

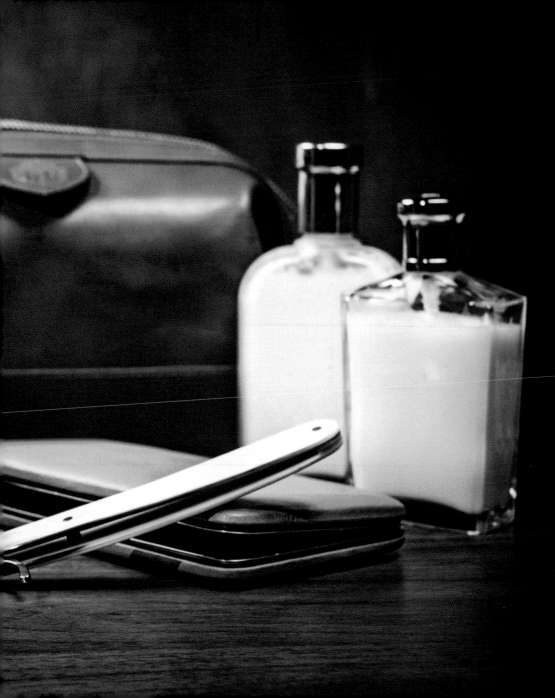

Hugh, on the other hand, has developed an equally fine palate for travel in a personal capacity, relishing trips with his family whenever his schedule allows. Here are five of his must-visit cities around the world – including Ireland's capital, of course – and the best spots to grab a drink with a view.

These hotels are within reach when they come courtesy of an international production company's budget, but more usually they are super-glam hotspots to visit for a cocktail and some celebrity spotting.

If you're in town, put on your finest attire and try these venues for a taste, however brief, of the high life.

ROME: PALAZZO MANFREDI

When it comes to views of Rome, it doesn't get much better than this hotel, which overlooks the Colosseum from its incomparable terrace.

PARIS: FOUR SEASONS HOTEL GEORGE V

This five-star hotel offers a grand setting with unrivalled views of the City of Lights, and its adequately named 'Le Bar' is a luxurious hideaway from the bustling streets of Paris.

NEW YORK: MR PURPLE

This property encapsulates flamboyant sophistication in the heart of the Big Apple – and indulging in the delights of its cocktail menu won't require you to remortgage your home.

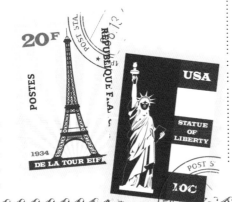

TOKYO: HYATT REGENCY

Should you ever find yourself in this part of the world, the Hyatt is a must-visit, even for a quick glass of Pinot Noir. Its rooftop swimming pool (on the 52nd floor no less) is internationally renowned, and the elevator – featured in *Lost in Translation* – will trigger some serious social media envy.

LOS ANGELES: FOUR SEASONS BEVERLY WILSHIRE

Chances are, at the table next to you, there'll be a deal being struck for a new franchise, new signing or some other A-list business. And if you can afford the eye-watering cost of a night's stay, you'll also be treated to complementary use of the 'house car' in the exquisite form of a Rolls-Royce Phantom.

DUBLIN: SOPHIE'S AT THE DEAN

This new-on-the-scene hotel is one of Ireland's few rooftop venues, offering the city's ultimate chill-out space, along with a commitment to combining old-world décor with modern service.

When travelling to a new city that doesn't speak your native language, learn a few useful, friendly phrases to show your appreciation of their culture and mother tongue. It is good to talk – and you will leave a lasting impression of you as an individual and as a representative of your nation.

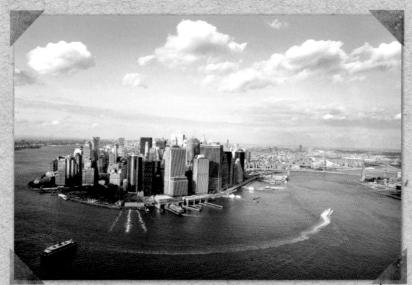

The Big Apple – as awe-inspiring as ever!

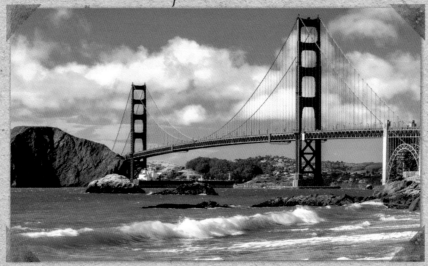

There may not be a heaven, but there is San Francisco . . .

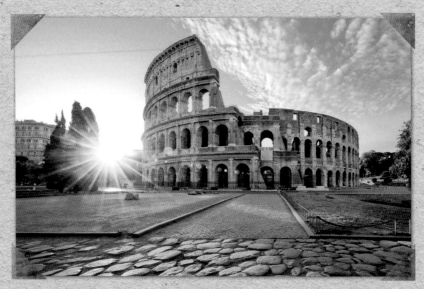

All roads lead to Rome - visiting the Colosseum.

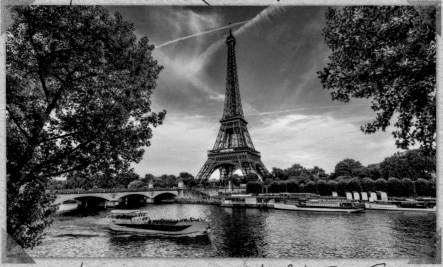

Living the dream on the banks of the River Seine.

The shores of etiquette

Everyone loves a beach holiday, but don't let your standards or your towel slip whether you're surfing or sunbathing. Steer clear of these sun-kissed faux pas.

☞ *The beach is a place to relax. No one will be pleased if you bring noisy music, set up camp too close to your neighbours and engage in boisterous games of frisbee or football.*

☞ *However hot it is, there's no excuse for swimming trunks on the skimpy side of skimpy. You are not Borat and probably not Daniel Craig either.*

☞ *When you leave the beach, beach wear ceases to be appropriate. Cover up for that trip to the shop or a restaurant.*

☞ *Don't turn into a lobster. It's not very stylish.*

☞ *And always leave the beach at least as tidy as you found it – take all your stuff away.*

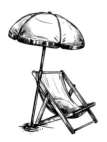

Hair-raising travel

Maybe you fancy a VIP barber treatment while away from home? Here's the Grafton Barber's insider nod on the finest barbershops the world has to offer.

THE NED IN LONDON, ENGLAND

One of London's newest high-end hotels and members' clubs features a speakeasy-style barbershop for guests and non-guests alike, offering traditional wet shaves and facials.

GENTLEMAN'S TONIC AT ATLANTIS, THE PALM IN DUBAI

In the United Arab Emirates, luxury reigns supreme. At the Atlantis Hotel, a venue frequented by international travellers, the in-house barbershop offers everything from a beard trim to the 45-minute 'Royal Shave', a truly indulgent treatment.

BALI BARBER IN BALI, INDONESIA

Ideal for any expat, tourist or traveller, this world-class barbershop blends American barbering traditions with Indonesian hospitality to create an experience like no other. On offer is an exclusive range of services from spa treatments to Cuban cigars, with great music and even greater customer care creating a truly vibrant backdrop.

ASTOR PLACE HAIRSTYLISTS IN MANHATTAN, NEW YORK

A true New York legend. Founded in 1947 with just five chairs, Astor Place is now the city's biggest barbershop and salon. Everyone from A-list celebs, world-class musicians, tourists and locals can enjoy – and afford – the charm of downtown New York when they step through the doors of this landmark salon. Staff speak Spanish, French, Polish, Russian and more – and have extraordinary tales to tell of clients ranging from billionaires to the city's elected officials and film stars.

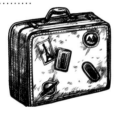

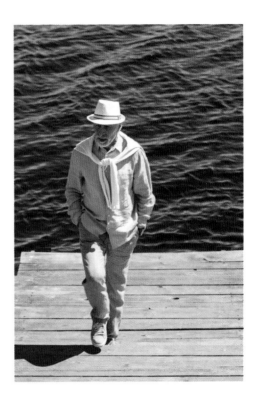

CUTTING REMARKS

'One's destination is never a place,
but always a new way of seeing things.'

Wise words indeed, from American novelist Henry Miller. Travel is an opportunity to further yourself and see the world through someone else's eyes, to educate yourself about the wider world and to spread the principles of gentlemanliness to every destination you visit. And if you have the opportunity to enjoy some luxury in the process, so be it!

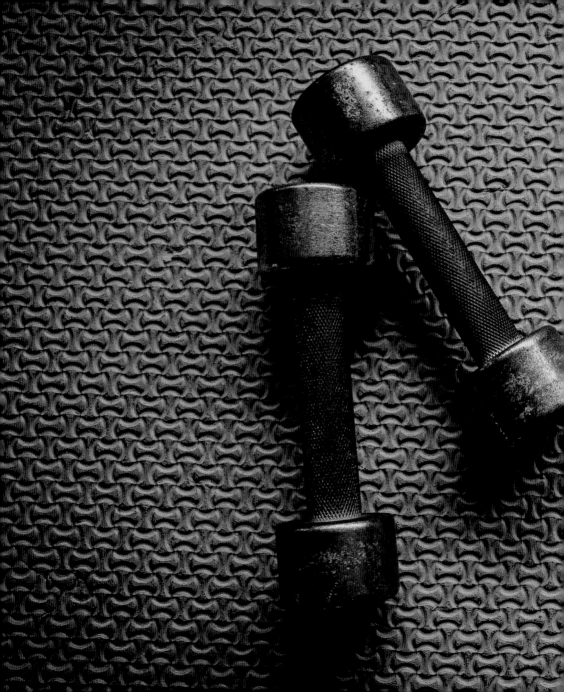

CHAPTER 9
Working Out

"Knowledge is knowing that a tomato is a fruit. Wisdom is knowing not to put it in a fruit salad." — Brian O'Driscoll, quoting Miles Kington

Exercising the Gentlemanly Way

THE PRINCIPLES OF BEING A gentleman apply to all aspects of life and your gym is no exception. Like most social situations, there is a series of unwritten rules which require focus if you are to be part of the communal culture, and also thrive at personal challenges, develop new friendships and achieve individual goals.

There's something invigorating about the ritual of exercise and its trappings. It acts as a haven for like-minded people, most of whom are there to focus on achieving their personal best, peppered with a healthy dose of competition. With that, comes a responsibility to maintain civility and respect for others' physical activity, which can be especially difficult to remember during those times when your testosterone is rising and heart rate is pumping.

This book is brimming with advice on grooming, and it's clearly the case that good grooming builds on emotional and physical wellbeing. Fitness levels play an intrinsic role in creating – and maintaining – a sense of purpose, strength and achievement that's rooted deep in one's character.

How to exercise smart

A devotion to fitness doesn't have to be an all-encompassing lifestyle decision, especially if your schedule isn't one that permits you as much free time as you'd like, but there are easy ways to cultivate the glow of physical health as part of your day-to-day life.

In a world whose view is increasingly channelled towards the digital, it's easy to subscribe to the many fitness-related online options for inspiration and advice. If it appeals to you, there is more practical and spiritual information available than ever before about exercise and its seemingly endless benefits.

THE ONLY BAD WORKOUT IS NO WORKOUT

You may be blessed with a fast metabolism or be someone who has to push that extra mile to satisfy your goals and maintain your weight, but even the smallest bouts of exercise can improve your overall fitness levels.

The freedom of discipline

The discipline of a gym habit is a near-guarantee of personal growth – you push yourself, you learn limits and work towards goals. The freedom of increased confidence, emotional health and significant boosts to your energy levels acts as a real motivation.

If you're just retuning to – or starting afresh with – an exercise regime, be patient. You won't see results overnight, especially if you're over the age of 25. But here are a few eminently doable tips to motivate you.

How to kick start your fitness habit

SET REALISTIC GOALS. *Like any new challenge, it's important to remember that you're standing at the bottom of your own proverbial mountain. Be patient with your progress, but stay on top of your game. If possible, set up a monthly appointment with a personal trainer you trust and who you feel 'gets you' in terms of your fitness aspirations. You can work with them to confirm your measurements, monitor progress and boost your routine in order to give yourself a fresh start.*

GET UP EARLIER. *Even if it's only by half an hour. It's a well-known secret of successful people that they like to begin their daily routines with exercise to clear the mind and welcome the day with joy. Whether it's 50 lengths of the pool, a few laps of your local park, a buzz-generating circuits session or a series of sun salutations, starting the day with physical activity is life-transforming.*

MAKE SURE YOU'RE COMFORTABLE. *There's little point in signing up somewhere you won't feel encouraged or confident as you progress. Like anything, listen to your instincts – and be bold enough to walk away if an environment doesn't work for you.*

TRY A PERSONAL TRAINER.

In this day and age, a personal trainer is no longer a luxury exclusively afforded to Hollywood's elite, rather it's an essential service provided at most gyms. If you want to go the extra mile, sign up for a service that you can visit at specific intervals. Most trainers offer a package deal for regular customers and for those who pay up front. Classes can be a good, cost-effective approach too, if you find one to fit your schedule and interests.

DOWNLOAD IT.

There are a multitude of apps to track your food intake and steps for the day. They will help keep note of your calories, and can analyse your diet against goals you set at sign-up. Fitbits can be a great accessory to record your steps and activity throughout the day, but there are also apps you can download for free for instant, and economical, assistance.

MAKE IT A FRIENDS' GAME.

Find a friend, colleague or neighbour to factor in some exercise with. Not only can you enjoy a discounted personal training session for two, you'll find yourself more motivated to hit the gym alongside a friend. Pretty soon, you'll have no problem visiting without them. Clubs – football, running, boxing, cycling – are the perfect tried-and-tested way to maximise your fitness and enjoyment when it comes to training, competing and excelling at your chosen sport.

REMEMBER THE BENEFITS.

The gains from exercise are endless: weight loss, improved sleep and general health, and a renewed libido (not least because resistance training increases testosterone). And, as is well documented, the positive impact of exercise on mental health is remarkable – there's nothing better for an invigorating boost to self-esteem, mental clarity and feelings of vitality and joie de vivre. You mightn't always be in the mood to get your gear on and make that trek to the gym – or out the front door for a run or cycle – but remember, 'If it's worth having, it's worth working for.'

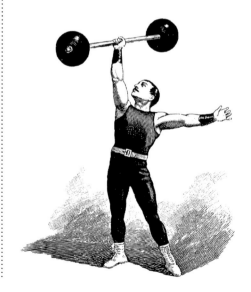

Don't be a Gym Rat: Part 1

Hugh has decades of gym time under his belt. His must-follow rules will ensure you're sending the right message, especially if you're new to the gym.

READ THE RULES. *Every environment has its own set of guidelines for members to abide by. They are rarely ground-breaking, but remember them and be sure to follow them. They're there for a reason.*

WIPE DOWN THE EQUIPMENT. *While you're working up a sweat, so has your machine and no one wants to use a machine with someone else's perspiration on it. Carry a towel with you so you can wipe yourself down too.*

STRETCH. *This is an important rule for you as an individual. Learn what is most appropriate for your body type and workout, and be sure to stretch before and after.*

DON'T HOG ANY MACHINE/WEIGHTS. *Unless you work unsociable hours and you tend to work out during off-peak times, chances are there is always somebody eyeing up something you're using. Be respectful of other people's time, which means you shouldn't take extended breaks anywhere but the locker room. Only use one set of weights at a time and don't monopolise them. Don't encroach on other people's space either – no one will appreciate you hanging around 'waiting' for them to finish.*

BE RESPECTFUL IN YOUR ATTITUDE. *If a woman is using weights don't presume she needs less time or lighter weights than you – and certainly don't offer her any unsolicited attention or 'advice'. In fact, apply this rule to everyone using the gym alongside you.*

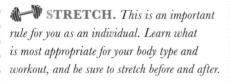

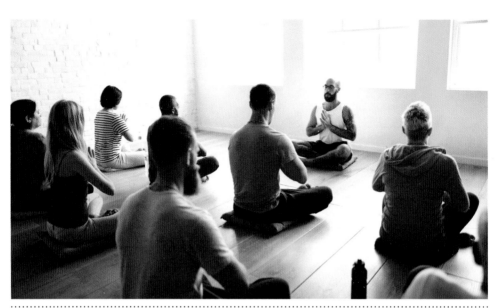

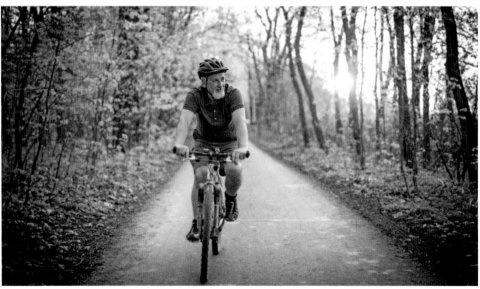

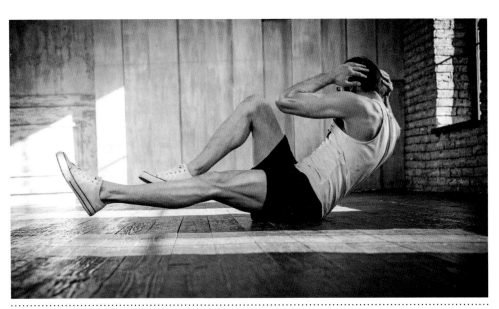

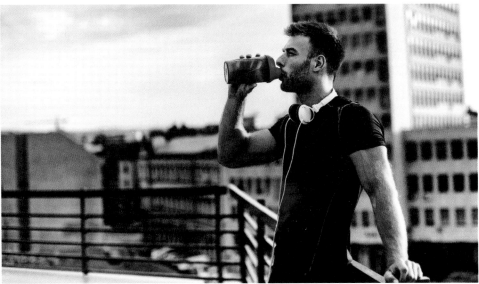

Don't be a Gym Rat: Part 2

RETURN WEIGHTS. *It sounds simple, but remember that if you wouldn't leave it out at home, you shouldn't leave it out somewhere else. Put any equipment you use back where you found it. Not least because you might be able to lift something the size of a truck, but perhaps the next person along would prefer not to.*

WATCH YOUR NOISES. *There's no need for excessive grunting in any situation.*

BEWARE OF YOUR PERSONAL HYGIENE *– even before the gym. You want to provide a pleasant environment for other members and staff, and if you're a little pungent after a particularly warm day, shower before you go in order to ensure you don't make anyone else feel uncomfortable.*

DRESS APPROPRIATELY. *The increase in availability of athleisure ranges for men and women around the world means there is more variety than ever before across all budgets. Try them. But don't go overboard on the branded sportswear. The gym isn't a catwalk to showcase your lucrative sponsorship deal, but neither is it an opportunity to wear out your skankiest T-shirts and shorts. There comes a time when even the hottest wash won't cut it: all fitness clothing is destined for the great laundry basket in the sky.*

WATCH YOUR SOCIAL MEDIA ACTIVITY. *There's nothing wrong with taking a selfie in the gym, but never include someone else in the background. Nobody wants to be caught unawares and red-faced in a stranger's picture.*

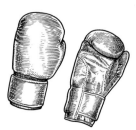

Will swimmers kindly refrain from . . .

Michael Phelps, the most decorated Olympic athlete of all time, has a thing or two to say about pool etiquette. And he might be an exception to the rule that the practice of industry leaders should be followed – namely for his stance on . . . relieving yourself during a swim session.

'I think everybody pees in the pool,' he says. 'It's kind of a normal thing to do for swimmers. When we're in the pool for two hours, we don't really get out to pee.'

It's a slightly off-putting reality to be confronted with, but chlorine really does kill the subsequent germs. Aside from his lax approach to in-pool hygiene, you might like to follow Phelps's system of self-belief, if not his gruelling training schedule. He says that his coach, Bob Bowman, worked to take the word 'can't' out of his vocabulary:

'So that I could broaden my mind and believe that I could do whatever I wanted to. And I think that was a big key of us being so successful. I was always a kid or a young man that would think as big as I could possibly think. And dream as big as I could possibly dream.'

BE A CLASS ACT

For most new skills, classes are required to familiarise yourself with what it is you're trying to acheive, so follow these three non-negotiable rules to ensure everyone in your space, including you, has the most satisfying class possible.

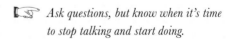 *Show up on time. Always.*

Ask questions, but know when it's time to stop talking and start doing.

Don't make excuses. If you're there, give it 100%.

Beyond the gym

The gym isn't the only place to reap the benefits of physical exercise. We checked in with some sports devotees about the etiquette that governs their particular passions.

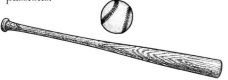

RUNNING – this is a super simple, back-to-basics workout that can be done by just about anyone anywhere. Buy yourself a decent pair of trainers from a specialist running shop and off you go. But . . .

⚜ *Be competitive, but know your limits. If you're racing, it's best not to elbow your way to the very front of the start line. You're not Sir Mo Farah and you'll annoy (and trip up) the serious athletes.*

⚜ *When you're out for a sunny Sunday session, be civil. Nod or say hello to your fellow runners and step out of the path of ambling toddlers and dog walkers with grace.*

⚜ *You might need to spit the phlegm from your mouth or nose. But not in front of anyone else. Please.*

SWIMMING – if you want to swim seriously for fitness, then it's worth taking lessons to ensure your technique is spot-on.

⚜ *Your local pool can be a haven of chloriney peacefulness. Don't disturb it by thrashing up and down like a beast. If you're training for Ironman or similar, join a club of like-minded folk.*

⚜ *Never grumble or push your way past if someone in the lane is slower than you – wait, overtake at the end and say thank you.*

CYCLING – all you really need is a decent bike to reap the benefits – and the leg muscles – of this classic sport.

⚜ *As oft-maligned road users, cyclists are hyper-alert to etiquette, so give your sport a good name. Be a decent human being – don't shout abuse, make obscene gestures, cut people up or think that red traffic light doesn't apply to you.*

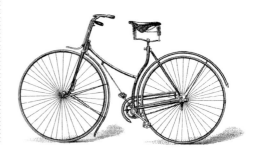

❧ Learn how to maintain your bike – or at least send it for a regular service. As you would with your car, clean it. A bike that's not well looked after is noisy, dangerous and a hazard to others. If you see a fellow cyclist struggling with a breakdown, why not stop and help?

YOGA – all you need for yoga is your personal strength, a commitment to achieving your goals – and a yoga mat. But it's worth signing up for a class to get expert one-on-one guidance.

❧ Not only is yoga a great weight loss aid and natural strength builder, it's practised by athletes worldwide including Irish rugby legend Brian O'Driscoll, NFL superstar Tom Brady and, of course, David Beckham. Yoga increases flexibility,

muscle tone and offers incomparable boosts to self-awareness and mental health.

❧ Men are a dime a dozen in yoga classes, so don't let gender stop you from trying. Patience is key, especially if it's your first time stretching your body in this way – be prepared for it to take several months before you notice real physical change. At first, stay at the back of the class and observe the pros in all their glory.

*❧ Always bring a towel with you – one to put on your mat and one to wipe your sweat away (you don't want those cross **contaminating**).*

❧ Being quiet is the greatest gift you can give to your classmates, so connect with your inner chakra while shaping your body in new and exciting ways.

CUTTING REMARKS

Sport isn't just about physical benefits. It also provides the satisfaction of personal achievement, the structure of a meaningful schedule and the sense of camaraderie that comes with being part of a team. And the true joy is that you are never too old to start! But do get checked out first if your health or age demands it.

• • •

Feelings of inadequacy can be our biggest hurdle on the road to physical fitness, but have you ever heard of anyone regretting a visit to the gym? Probably not. But you will have experienced regret at not pushing yourself towards a path of physical fitness. Listen to Michael Phelps: self-belief marks the start of that journey.

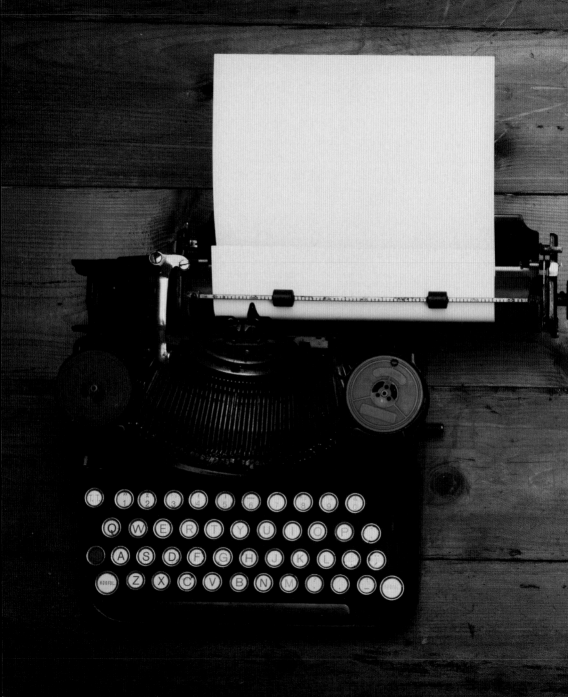

CHAPTER 10
In Real Life

"The less you know, the more you believe." – Bono

Social Media

IT'S A LITTLE ON THE NOSE TO point out that many of our modern interactions are digitised rather than taking the form of face-to-face conversations. But it's clearly true that your online persona is nearly as important as your real-life presence.

Social media activity is often the first port of call for a future opportunity, whether it be a potential employer or a more personal love interest. It isn't just a place to show off as you live-your-best-life, but it's also a marker to the future while providing a link to your past, connecting you with former classmates, long-lost family members and others who share your interests, however eclectic.

In recent years, skilled practitioners, be they chefs, architects, lifestyle gurus or fashion commentators have risen to the top of their profession to become sought-after celebrities. Many of these creative people have used high-level social media savvy to drive awareness of their personal 'brand', which in turn has significantly enhanced their influence – and earning ability.

INTERNETIQUETTE

Your behaviour online should remain at least as civil and purposeful as it would in real life. This requires a distinct 'internetiquette' – which isn't to say you can't have fun, but it is to say that you should be considerate and respectful.

The Grafton Barber's social media channels all provide direct connections with existing, new and potential customers. A small team has the task of bringing the spirit of the Grafton Barber to life online, key to which is a deep appreciation for the communities in which the barbers have worked for the past 40 years.

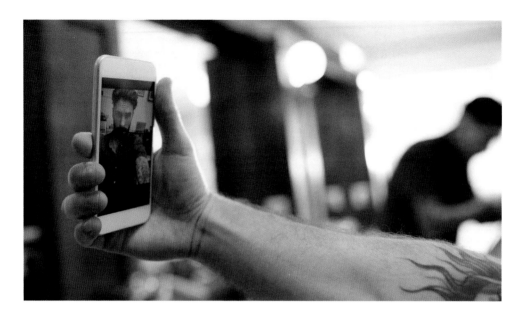

Circles of goodwill

Integration into every location in which a new Grafton Barber store opens is vital. Store managers are encouraged to join the local chamber of commerce and establish links with charities and groups to show commitment to their new community.

The real-life goodwill created by this philanthropy creates a beneficial circle that rewards all involved, making the new store a positive contribution to local lives.

'We try to think globally and act locally,' the digital team says. 'The ethos of the Grafton Barber's virtual presence isn't unlike that of its real-life partner: the personalities of the two work hand in hand. We want to achieve the same universal ethos across our brand. It's one which portrays the principles of being a gentleman to our digital visitors.'

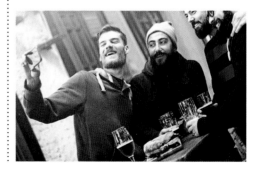

The 10 Digital Commandments

1 POST REGULARLY, but not too frequently. Your content is not nearly as interesting to the wider world as you think. Every platform has different expectations, but as a rule of thumb, post a maximum of three times a day on Instagram, once a fortnight on YouTube, twice a week on Facebook and as much as you like on Twitter. Updates are essential to build a following, but you'll find more people clicking 'unfollow' if you're clogging their newsfeeds with unnecessary verbiage or poor quality content.

2 DON'T COMPLAIN about your job. Your personal accounts are not a place to gripe about frustrations you may have, and there are documented cases of people being fired over their social media posts. Educate yourself on your workplace's policy before posting.

3 DON'T OVERSHARE. Celebrities use social media to project the 'normal' side of their lives: cooking at home, playing with their children or watching their favourite TV shows. It's part of a carefully choreographed business model to appeal to a wide audience, something that isn't required for the rest of us. My guess is you're not a celebrity, in which case the oversharing of personal information becomes irritating for friends and followers and has the opposite effect to that intended.

4 DON'T ASK FOR FOLLOWERS. It comes across as desperate. Instead, identify a niche area where you can assimilate your work. Most platforms are oversaturated, so do your research and determine exactly where you should fit. Be careful not to overuse hashtags as it's seen as poor 'internetiquette'.

5 ALWAYS ENGAGE WITH FOLLOWERS. If you are a business owner or a private individual racking up some social mileage, take the time to interact with the people who got you there. If someone comments, respond promptly. It's a mark of respect. It will also encourage others to get to know you.

6 CENSOR YOURSELF. If you wouldn't say it in conversation at work, then don't say it online where the entire world can access it now and for evermore.

7 DON'T BOAST. The 'influencer' market, comprised of 'ordinary' people who happen to live fabulously lavish and beautifully curated lives, is a heavily populated one. Step away from bragging about your accomplishments, no matter how tempting it may be, or how proud you are. It's an easy way to alienate friends, family and followers.

8 BE HONEST and offer something of value. There's no harm in filtering a picture slightly, but to FaceTune yourself beyond recognition is a no-no; as is hyperbolising your skills or talents. Honesty is always the best policy, but know when to rein it in. If you're growing a following, identify your message and don't be a needle in a haystack. People will always follow someone interesting; you need to figure out what it is about you that will engage others.

9 ALWAYS CHECK your spelling and grammar. Mistakes are deeply frustrating to see from the outside; all your posts require is a quick proofread to ensure a more streamlined, professional appearance.

10 DON'T FORGET that real-life rules apply to your online existence: being behind a screen doesn't actually afford you anonymity, especially when you have something critical to say. Always think before you post, then read – and read again. The golden rule is: if you wouldn't say it to someone's face, it's best to keep your thoughts to yourself.

PS THE 2 A.M. RULE states that nothing good happens after that hour in the morning . . . And it goes without saying that posting under the influence is particularly hazardous.

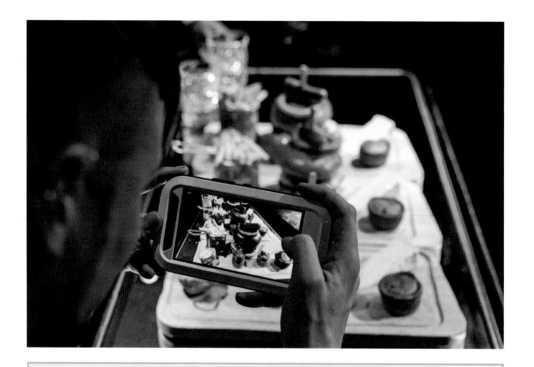

CUTTING REMARKS

Smart phones and accessible technology might be the cornerstone of our communications, but still – nothing beats real life. Steve Jobs said it best: 'Your time is limited, so don't waste it living someone else's life.' Granted, he meant this in terms of self-belief – 'Don't let the noise of others' opinions drown out your own inner voice' – but the principle applies to your life online too.

• • •

Know when to put the phone down for a digital detox – whether it lasts a few minutes, an hour, a day or even longer. Don't forget your real life – with real people, real conversation and, most valuable of all, real memories.

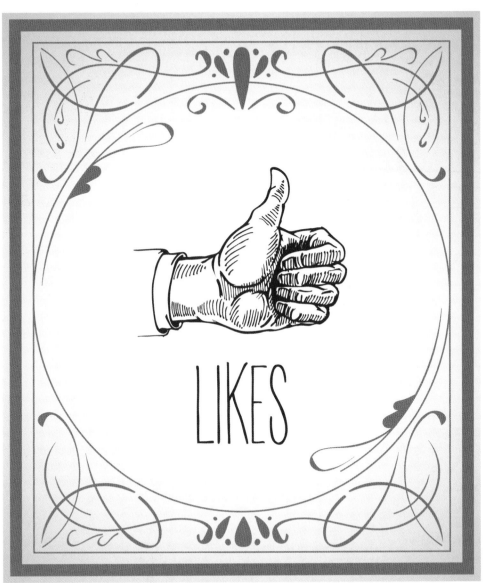

LIKES

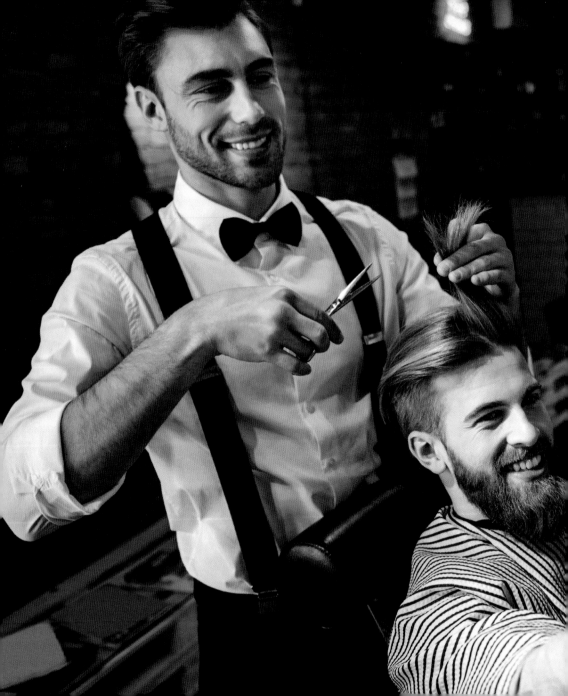

CHAPTER 11

Schmooze it or Lose it

"I kept telling myself this word, process. Focus on my process, don't care about the result."

– Rory McIlroy

Networking

THE FOUNDATION OF EVERY BRAND is built on connections – connections that may come in the form of customers, colleagues or friends. With such an illustrious clientele, the McAllisters have clearly mastered the art of networking through natural charm and a world-renowned skill set. In any one day, each may deal with 20 individual customers, so the capacity to lead engaging conversation is invaluable.

As two of Ireland's most successful businessmen, reaching every corner of the country through their salons and employing more than 200 staff, few are as well positioned to offer advice on the cornerstones of networking – which they see as simple sociability and good grace.

With an inner circle that reads like the guestlist at a major awards ceremony, it's fair to say that the brothers are arguably two of Ireland's best networkers. The key to their success is rooted in pragmatism, charisma and self-acceptance – and a disregard for the niceties of social climbing.

In many traditional workplaces camaraderie can build naturally over time between employees. But when you're the owner of a business which sees hundreds of customers a day, each of whom expects the same individualised VIP treatment, an ability to bond naturally and with genuine warmth is essential. Enduring success is thanks to the loyalty of thousands of 'regular' customers.

'We're friends with people from all walks of life,' Hugh says. 'It's important you don't forget yourself. As a wise man once said, always be nice to people on the way up, because sometimes you'll meet them on the way down.'

TALENT SHOWS

As business owners, the McAllisters' networks are pleasingly blurred, but they trust that talent and dedication, like cream, will always rise to the top.

• • •

'A network will grow organically if you're good at what you do and you're in the right profession,' Conor says. 'Passion, competence and a willingness to learn and share will stand you in good stead.'

Fake it till you make it

Self-confidence is a skill. Here are some simple techniques you can adopt to boost your sense of value, and help you feel at ease when building your networks.

☞ UNDERSTAND BODY LANGUAGE. *Identify a cue for welcome conversation and for when it's time to walk away. Everyone remembers someone who couldn't take a hint and lingered too long chatting.*

☞ IF YOU BUILD IT, THEY WILL COME. *Visualise your goals and identify ways of making them happen. If you are looking for a new* job *then directly contact the individual in charge and don't be afraid to ask an expert for advice. Playing to someone's ego in asking for advice is one of the most often neglected ways of picking someone's brains.*

☞ DON'T BE TOO HARD ON YOURSELF. *If your dream job – or partner – is taking longer than you thought to come into your life, take a step back to self-reflect. If there's something more you could be doing, roll up your sleeves and do it. If things take more time to click, be patient and realise not everything in life is in your control.*

☞ PRACTISE AFFIRMATIONS. *It sounds cheesy, but motivational speakers around the world will preach the value of self-belief and praise. The power of positive thinking should never be underestimated and remember – whatever it is, if you put the time and energy in, you are worthy.*

The boundaries of our lives are ever blurring, but the je ne sais quoi that makes you you is something any prospective employer, partner or friend will notice straight away. You may not realise how your transferable skills can translate into a work context. For example, are you a middle child? Chances are you're an expert in mediation and conflict resolution.

Five easy ways to maximise your own personal network

1 SAY YES AND FIGURE OUT THE REST LATER. If it's good enough for Richard Branson, it's good enough for the rest of us. Identify an opportunity when it comes your way and, while you should always be aware of what you're aligning your personal brand with, grab every worthwhile chance with both hands.

- - - - - - - -

2 BE NICE TO EVERYONE. Kindness isn't just a virtue, it's a practice. Always treat everyone from the host of the party to the server with the same consideration and respect.

- - - - - - - -

3 KEEP YOUR FEET ON THE GROUND. Remain humble and grounded, regardless of how successful you become. You never know how long you will be lucky enough to remain at the top and it's important to stay level-headed in all aspects of your life.

4 LEARN HOW TO HANDLE DIFFICULT PEOPLE AND TRICKY SITUATIONS. Conor recalls dealing with a particular actor during the filming of *Space Truckers*. The actor insisted on having a mirror on set so he could check himself for every scene. Conor put his expertise as a hairstylist to good use so as to overcome this awkward scenario. He also made sure to try and understand why the actor was so frustrated. Show a challenging personality how talented you are and let them know what is and isn't an acceptable in a work environment.

- - - - - - - -

5 GET CREATIVE. You are the only person responsible for your own growth and you need to make opportunities happen by setting goals and practical ways to achieve them. Enquire directly with an employer about job prospects instead of waiting for a formal ad or, if appropriate, host an event to showcase your skills.

Enhancing your digital network

How do you stand out in a world with infinite options? It's naïve to think that your ability alone will be enough to catch someone's eye, whether that someone is a potential employer, employee, partner or friend. Given that your digital persona is an extension of your real-life self, it's vital to educate yourself on how to effectively represent yourself online.

 YOU NEED AN ONLINE PRESENCE. *You don't need to be a web developer or be fluent in HTML to plan your digital journey. First, you need to identify what it is you're trying to achieve – are you looking for your dream job or are you setting up a dating profile? Truthfully, they are not so dissimilar – on a date and at a job interview you share personal information, goals and show your true self, and it's no bad thing to extend this online. Be honest, but selective too. Familiarise yourself with all the different, relevant options and build slowly.*

GET SOCIAL MEDIA SAVVY. *Ask for advice from your friends, children or read about new techniques and websites to give yourself a competitive edge. On LinkedIn, for example, ensure you have a new, professionally relevant photo and that your resumé is regularly updated with fresh achievements and snappy endorsements. The golden rule is: never lie. If you hyperbolise your skillset,*

you'll be found out pretty quickly and no one likes to feel like they've been had.

UPSKILL. *Don't be afraid to sign up to a real-life course in digital media to get to the nitty-gritty of effective online communication. Most cities have weekend or evening classes and staying ahead of the curve can be fun – and it's always better than simply keeping up.*

NO PRESSURE

Of course, it can sometimes feel hard to stay afloat in an ever-changing world, regardless of your industry or personal predilections, but confidence and a cool head will never fail you.

There's lots to be said for an ability to remain focused under pressure, to be willing to compromise and get the job done. And you can be certain that people around you will always rank those personality traits as among the most precious you have to offer.

How to handle those awkward social situations

☞ **KEEP A COOL HEAD.** *Never respond to aggression with more aggression, this only exacerbates a situation. Instead, listen to what the person is saying and try to find the root cause of their frustration. Oftentimes, listening to someone's grievances, and letting them know you're trying to understand their point of view, is enough to take the heat out of a potentially volatile situation.*

☞ **CHECK YOUR BODY LANGUAGE.** *You can generate empathy and rapport with another by using gestures, tone of voice and eye contact that are open genial and polite rather than hostile or provoking. Relax and smile, it's often as simple as that!*

☞ **DON'T BE AFRAID TO STAND UP FOR YOURSELF.** *While it's important to be open to compromise, there is no need to become someone else's doormat. Listen to a point, but if the conversation turns abusive, simply tell someone the conversation is over and you can resume when they've cooled off.*

☞ **BUT DON'T INSIST ON WINNING AT ALL COSTS.** *Sometimes the truly assertive course of action is to concede another's point of view with good grace.*

☞ **DEFUSE WITH HUMOUR.** *The judicious use of gentle, well-meaning wit is a brilliant diplomatic tool.*

☞ **WHEN IN DOUBT, WALK AWAY.** *This can often prove the toughest, but it's important to know when a conversation is going nowhere. In most cases, when things become heated, both parties benefit from taking a break, instead of repeating their frustrations over and over.*

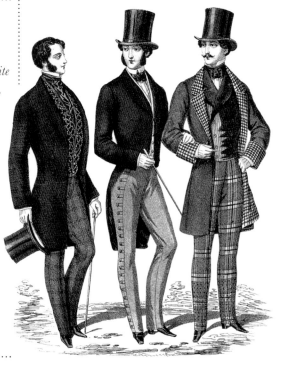

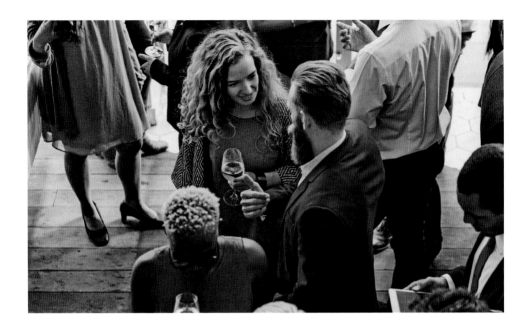

CUTTING REMARKS

Walt Bettinger, the CEO of international investment company Charles Schwab, identifies the value of personality traits in a professional environment and has a unique hack for getting down to it during the hiring process. He takes a candidate for breakfast and, beforehand, asks the server to give his prospect the wrong order in order to see how they handle it.

'I do that because I want to see how the person responds,' Bettinger says. 'That will help me understand how they deal with adversity. Are they upset, are they frustrated, or are they understanding? Life is like that, and business is like that. It's just another way to get a look inside their heart rather than their head.'

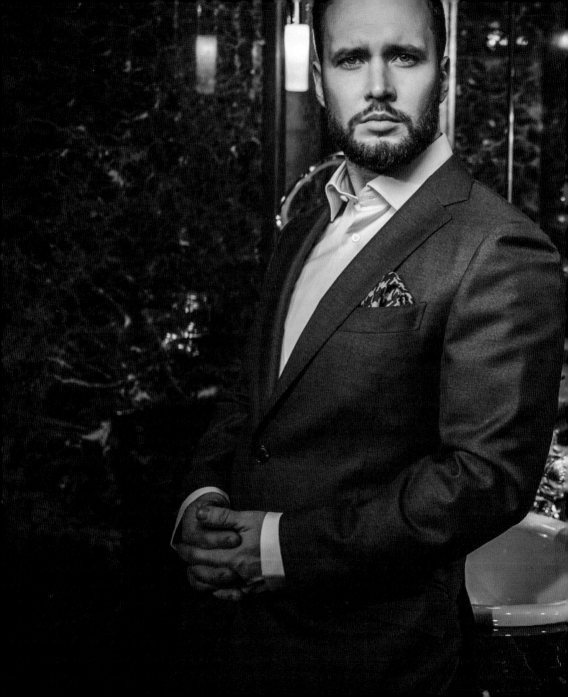

CHAPTER 12

The Grafton Barber Gentleman

"To learn one must be humble. But life is the great teacher." – James Joyce

The New Chivalry

WHO IS THE GRAFTON BARBER GENTLEMAN? He is someone committed to genuine chivalry in the modern world. He values classic conversation, polite interaction and one-on-one time with those closest to him. His preferred traits are courtesy, consideration and thoughtfulness – and he might just have a taste for the finer things in life! But he's an excellent friend too, someone who understands the value of relationships in his life, whether they are personal or professional.

Dating

To remain true to its proper meaning, chivalry may need some contemporary adjustments. When does chivalry become outdated or condescending – think, the dreaded mansplaining of a menu on a first date – and when does it become integral to establishing a connection of mutual respect? 'New chivalry' is a modern take on old-fashioned ideals, one which respects another's boundaries and independence, while also demonstrating a willingness to make someone special . . . well, feel special.

Modern dating can be tricky, but mutual courtesy will never go out of style.

Jumping off points

☞ **MAKE THE FIRST MOVE.**
There's nothing more attractive to a potential date than confidence. A confident man will know the right time to approach someone (and more importantly, the wrong time) with the right introduction. What might that be? Find some excuse to create the opportunity for small talk: if it's at a bar, order a drink at the same time and start conversation; in the gym, when you're putting

weights away; or if you're with a group of friends, find common ground to initiate a worthwhile conversation.

PICK UP THE PHONE. *Who doesn't like the flattery of being asked out on a date? If you meet someone you like, and think they feel the same, don't be afraid to call or ask them. If the conversation flows, ask them on an informal date – either for coffee or drinks. Both allow the opportunity for more conversation and so can determine your compatibility without the stuffiness of a dinner date.*

GO OFF-PISTE. *If you're feeling adventurous, give yourselves plenty to bond over by showing off your moves at the ice rink, getting all art buff at a local gallery, or catching some views at a scenic park nearby.*

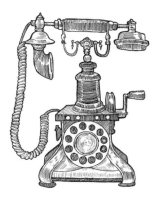

FORGET THE WAITING GAME. *Ignore everything the grapevine ever told you about the 'three day rule'. Yes, playing a little bit hard to get never hurt in building on those early-romance butterflies, but we live in an age of near-constant communication. If the date went well, let the person know the next day and allow an organic opportunity for a follow-up.*

First date faux pas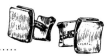

DON'T TALK ABOUT YOUR EX. *There is no excuse for speaking about past relationships on a first date. It tells your prospective partner that you're not over your ex (in which case, why are you dating?) and creates an uncomfortable atmosphere in which you are sharing an autopsy of your former love with a virtual stranger.*

NEVER BRING UP MONEY. *In the early days of a relationship – or a friendship as the case may be – speaking about your salary or financial ambitions is simply in bad taste. When it comes to the bill, always pay – at least on the first date. If it goes well, your date might like to pay for drinks afterwards, but 'Going Dutch' has no place on a chivalrous first date.*

AVOID POLITICS. *Politics is one of the most divisive topics any two people can discuss, even with an established connection. If both your*

personal passions play this way, then it can provide an exciting beginning to a satisfying relationship; but if, more often than not, analysing governmental idiocy evokes a certain ire within you, it's best to leave that subject to the second date.

⇒ CHAT-UP LINES ARE CHEESY.

Whoever said chat-up lines are the way to anyone's heart is woefully misguided. Nobody wants to hear about how they look as if they 'fell from heaven' or how they are 'the answer to all my prayers'. Be natural. Be honest. Be yourself.

⇒ DON'T COME ON TOO STRONG.

Even if you think you've found your soulmate, you must respect that the other person may not share those feelings and, as such, you should remain considerate in your communication. If you don't get a text back, take the hint and gracefully move on. Under no circumstances should you keep messaging – or, even worse, contacting them through other means. If there's a connection, you will both feel it and it will grow, unforced.

The motto of new chivalry

Chivalry isn't limited to dating, but can be incorporated into all aspects of your life, whether it's at work, home or during your commute.

A chivalrous man should always:

☞ Help an older – or not so much older – person with their bags if they are clearly struggling.

☞ Give up their seat on public transport for anyone who needs it – including people who are less able to stand, pregnant women and those with small children.

☞ Open the door for their partner on a date.

☞ Extend these courtesies to all those you interact with. Remember the rule which states: 'If someone is nice to you, but rude to the waiter, they are not a nice person.'

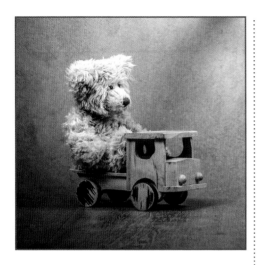

Hugh recalls his favourite holiday as a visit to Cushendall, near their home in Belfast, Northern Ireland. It's settled at the foot of Glenballyeamon, one of the nine Glens of Antrim. And these fond childhood memories have influenced everything from their business practices to their line of fragrances.

Neither claims to be a parenting guru, but they are ardent believers in listening closely to your heart and head when it comes to your family. Here they share some words of wisdom they try to live by.

Parenting

Conor and Hugh are dedicated family men. Hugh has been married to his wife Denise for 20 years and they have two daughters, while Conor and Juanita have been married for 18 years and also have two children. The McAllisters live in a rural Irish town outside Dublin, where their homes are directly across the road from one another, with their parents nearby too.

'We were lucky. We never wanted for love or the necessities of life,' Conor says. 'We're keen to replicate that for our children, as our childhood was one rooted in adventure. Our father could make anything exciting, even something like a day-trip to a neighbouring town.'

WHERE THE HEART IS

Both brothers aim to emulate the parenting style they experienced in their own childhoods, which they look back on with such affection. Like most parents, they do their utmost to foster a relaxed and happy home environment.

• • •

'Our mother is so protective and kind,' Hugh says. 'She has always been supportive of us – no one was ever allowed to criticise her children!'

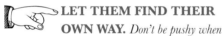
VALUE YOUR HEALTH.
As parents, the focus is on teaching the importance of commitment and fostering the teamwork that comes with sports or other extracurricular activities. Healthy eating is essential – but there's no need to go gluten, dairy and sugar-free unless your digestive system requires it. There's a lot to be said for a homemade dinner – and the fun of making it with everyone lending a helping hand.

LET THEM FIND THEIR OWN WAY. *Don't be pushy when it comes to your children's dreams – they might be different from yours. If they show a particular aptitude or talent, nurture it as best you can. Take a step back and remember they may not want to follow*

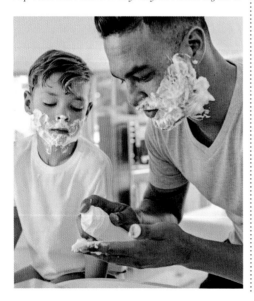

your footsteps into the family business. But if they do, don't sugar-coat the reality of what lies ahead.

HONESTY IS ALWAYS THE BEST POLICY. *Liars will always be caught out, whether their lies are of the big or the little white variety. Be truthful (and age appropriate) with your children and you and your family will benefit in spades. The child will grow up with a sense of assured confidence and trust, and you can sleep easy at night knowing you're raising them to be forthright with you and those around them.*

MAXIMISE QUALITY TIME. *Every parent's schedule is different: you may work shifts or be an at-home parent, but the case for quality time can never be made enough. This might be putting children to bed every night, establishing non-negotiable nightly (or weekly) family dinners, walks in the park or taking the bus together to football practice. Get to know your family afresh every day and you will all value those memories for ever.*

PASS ON AND CREATE TRADITIONS. *Family values vary from household to household, but there is something to be said for including manners, consideration and respect for your elders as part of day-to-day life in your home. There is no right or wrong way to do things, but fostering an environment of respect never goes out of fashion.*

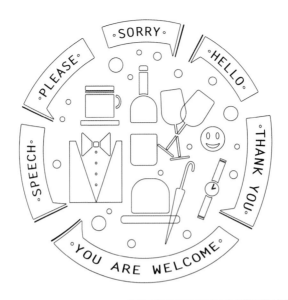

SORRY
PLEASE
HELLO
SPEECH
THANK YOU
YOU ARE WELCOME

⬩ ETIQUETTE ⬩

CUTTING REMARKS
Treat others the way you would like to be treated.
In theory, it sounds simple, in practice – life can be complicated. But this
straightforward mantra is key to long-lasting relationships in all aspects of your
life. Remembering it, especially during trying times,
will benefit you enormously.

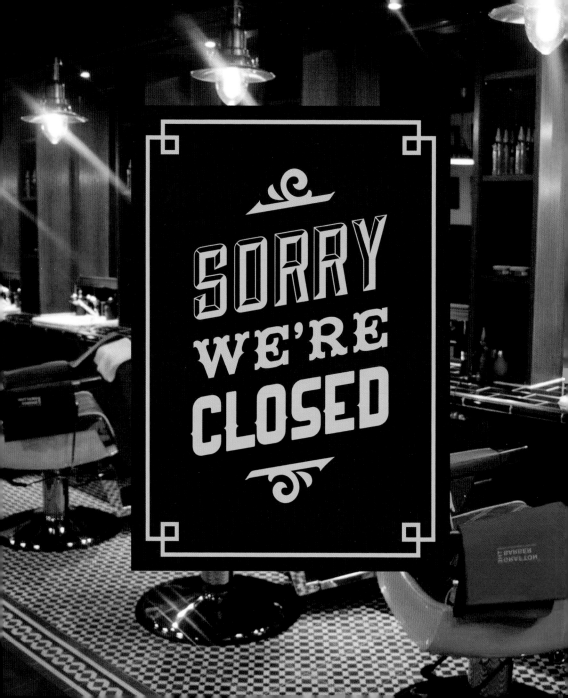

Meet the Grafton Barber Family

As business owners, Conor and Hugh have implemented a familial quality with all of their staff and customers. At present, all franchise owners of the 40-plus stores around Ireland are former staff members and the vast majority of their customers have been delighted to make use of their services for years. So, what makes the Grafton Barber so special?

In the words of customers

James Nelson, Celtic Tenor

I first met Hugh in the early days of my career (19 years ago!) when he styled me and other Celtic Tenors for the photoshoots for our first few albums. During our first shoot at Killua Castle in Co. Westmeath, Hugh was quite literally a tonic. Amid any stress or fatigue he had us laughing constantly – even by mistake when he complimented an octogenarian lady who made us tea by telling her she had 'lovely buns'!

Every photoshoot I have worked on is a happy memory because of the McAllister brothers. They are truly great guys to be around, but I cannot emphasise enough that they are the best at what they do. Our hair was always just right – but the jovial environment they created was invaluable.

They are a great advert for the Irish *Céad Míle Fáilte* (a hundred thousand welcomes), and they absolutely deserve their success. They are proof that hard work pays off. I like to think the Grafton Barber's success proves good karma really does exist!

Laurence Kinlan, Actor

I first met Conor in 2003 on the set of *Intermission*, a John Crowley film, where he was working as a hairdresser. At the time, I had hair down to my shoulders but I needed a skinhead look to play a ruffian that Colm Meaney had to chase through a block of flats. I warmed to Conor straightaway – not least of all because he has a strong Dublin accent like me! Since then, every time I go to Conor for a haircut, I treat him as an artist with me as the blank canvas. I completely trust him and let him do whatever he wants with my hair.

To see all their success, and how they have stayed so well grounded, is remarkable. It shows you that two brothers can work through anything. And it really is the two of them at the helm, even after all this time. They are witty, funny, smart – everything you want in a businessperson. I'm sure it's their personalities that have got them this far. They'd charm the ears off anyone they wanted to do business with!

John Fitzpatrick, Hotelier
I have been visiting the Grafton Barber on Grafton Street for more than 30 years, well before Hugh and Conor took over. Eddie McEvoy has been cutting my hair since then – he used to cut my father's hair, that's how long I've known him!

I've watched them transform the business from when they took over in 1994, incorporating old-fashioned ideals with a very modern touch. At the time, I had never seen anybody offer a coffee or a beer with a haircut or shave – it reminds me of the hospitality business, where your main concern is making sure everybody feels good. I especially appreciate how they treat Eddie and that mutual respect between him and the McAllisters.

What makes it so unique? They're a family business that works very, very well – there's no in-house fighting and the model has stood the test of time. It's a unique place, you can chat as long as you like, there's no rush. It really is special.

I live in New York and I will only let Eddie cut my hair when I return home every six weeks. That's how loyal I am!

In the words of franchise owners
Ginta Knizikeviciute, Dublin's Drumcondra, Co. Wicklow
When I moved to Ireland from Lithuania in 2006, I had no experience in cutting hair, but I was thrilled when I was offered a job as a trainee barber on Grafton Street – and I remained there for eight years.

I never anticipated how big it would become – at that time, there were four Grafton Barber shops in Ireland and now there are over 40. It's not like any barbershop I've ever known. The customer is always right – even when they're wrong! But it's that commitment to service that keeps customers coming back.

Hugh and Conor look after their business owners. In the beginning, I had no idea how to set up a business and they went through everything with me. They are both so hard-working. Often, when I finish for the day, they're still in the office and it's very telling that they encourage independent success with their staff by offering them franchises.

After so many years, it feels like one big family, not only with the business, but also in my personal life. I know that if I ever need anything, they will always be there.

Fabien Pollard, Dublin's International Financial Services Centre
Like many Irish people, I had been working in Australia before coming home in 2002. I began by working in the Grafton Barber in Arnotts department store and, within a year, they asked me to manage the new shop in the IFSC. In 2015, I jumped at the chance to purchase the franchise.

Before working with the McAllisters, I didn't know much about barbering. But as soon as I began work, I realised they had a very different attitude to customer service – it wasn't just about cutting hair, it was about making the customer feel extraordinary. I found myself becoming more articulate and really appreciating good manners. If you walk into a Grafton Barber anywhere, you will be met with a smile.

Did I ever think we'd be where we are now? Never. Am I surprised? Absolutely not. Hugh and Conor are proof that if you work hard and have a dream, you can make it happen. I believe that dream started the very first moment they opened the doors of their Grafton Street shop.

Peter Quinn, Dublin's Stillorgan
I first started working with the McAllisters in the mid 1990s when they opened their Grafton Street store. Then I left for a career in IT, but it didn't evoke that same sense of passion that barbering gave me. In 2014, my wife Tracy and I took the opportunity to buy a franchise.

The Grafton Barber is uniquely customer focused. So much so, that although our shop is very busy, we often don't hire new people because we're looking for a very specific type of person that fits the ethos of the brand – the career barber.

People ask what makes a good barber. I say, they have empathy with the client. They know what their customer is all about.

In the words of associates

John McKeown, Businessman
When I was MD of Beiersdorf Ireland Limited, we agreed a highly successful sponsorship arrangement with the Grafton Barber mobile unit in conjunction with the NIVEA for Men brand (now NIVEA Men).

When I met Conor to discuss the

sponsorship it came to light that his father Hugh had worked for my grandfather, also named John McKeown, who had a number of ladies and gents hairdressing shops and confectionery shops in Belfast. This felt surreal. It brought back great memories of visits to my grandfather's shops (particularly the confectionery ones!) when I was a child.

Hugh and Conor are both so full of energy, extremely hard working, dedicated and focused. The Grafton Barber is a model Irish success story built on a strong reputation for professionalism and first-class customer satisfaction. It highlights the success that an Irish company can achieve with a clear vision and strong branding.

Simon Delaney, Actor and writer
I met Conor on the set of *Bachelors Walk*, a TV series I starred in for RTÉ/BBC. Conor was our chief hairdresser, and from the first day on set, we clicked. I realised that Conor was at the top of his game, cutting and styling men's and women's hair on set, as per the director's instructions.

I then met Hugh, and Hugh Snr (the lads' dad, and the real power behind the throne!) on the set of *An Everlasting Piece*, a movie starring Billy Connolly and directed by Barry Levinson. The movie was based around Hugh Snr's life, and the tales from

his day as a hairdresser in Belfast during the Troubles. I've known the McAllister family now for almost two decades, and am proud to call them friends.

The lads are without doubt the hardest working people I've met. I've shared an office with them for five years, where I've watched them deal with the day-to-day running of their brand, as well as striving to stay ahead of the curve when it comes to innovations in barbering and men's grooming, constantly evolving the business to stay at the front, where they've been for over 20 years.

The Grafton Barber has become as well-known an Irish brand as Guinness and Riverdance. This is down to the boys' work ethic. You know that the Grafton Barber stands for excellence in barbering, customer service and quality of product. From the moment you walk into a salon, you know you're in safe hands. The Grafton Barber sets the standard not just in their particular field, but also in terms of how to run and grow a business. It's no surprise to me or anyone who knows the McAllister brothers that their brand is now the benchmark for barbering in Ireland. Watch this space.

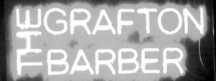

A final word by Saoirse Ronan

I first met Conor through my father when I was 13. My father Paul is also an actor and they had worked together on a film – and ever since Conor has been like an uncle to me. Both Conor and Hugh are hilarious, fun, supportive and kind.

They never stop talking – ever. Conor has kept me laughing for years and he is now a real part of my family. When Conor got me ready for the Irish premiere of *Brooklyn*, it was a really special night for the film and for me. I was glad we were all able to celebrate it together.

What the McAllisters have done with the Grafton Barber is to create a community for fathers and sons to visit their shops time and time again. Conor and Hugh have set the bar so high, for themselves and their team. There is a warmth and familiarity when you walk through the door.

The Grafton Barber is more than just a business – it's an extended family and it's the people that make it work. The more businesses that can offer that kind of genuine personal care, the better.

THANK YOUS

WE ARE FOREVER INDEBTED to our parents, Hugh and Bernadette McAllister, for such a happy upbringing, for an education in the school of life and for loving us the way you do.

Our wives, Denise and Juanita, who have stood by us through the crazy work hours, never questioning or doubting, but always supporting us. You have made our lives complete and we love you very much.

Now the trouble! Our children, who we are so proud of. We are here for them whatever journey they take in life. Elle, Amber, Pia and Max: we love you dearly.

Thanks to James Nesbitt for the best nights out; may they continue for an eternity. We are forever in your debt.

We've had the pleasure of watching Saoirse Ronan grow into a superstar. Thanks to you, and Monica and Paul Ronan, for being part of our family.

And our rollercoaster man, Simon Delaney. You are a great wingman in times good and bad. We both thank you again.

Other special thanks to:

Caitlin McBride, our brilliant co-author, John Fitzpatrick, Celtic Tenors – Matt, James and Daryl, Markus Feehily, Hugo McCollom, Laurence Kinlan, Colm McEvoy, Paul 'Ernest' Flynn, Paddy McKillan, Joe Ritchie, Siobhan Ronan, Saiva Pyneandee, Soudevi Cite, Lizzie McGhee, Jade Hanbury, Mark Rowe, Fabian Pollard, Jing Zheng, Antonio Evangilista, Mark Guider, Lisa Mallon, John Williams, Neringa Ratkelyte, Liam Egan, Victor Peiu, Gintare Knizikeviciute, Barry Whitelaw, Peter and Tracy Quinn, James Walsh, John O'Dowd, Vinil and Monica Kaveri, Jolanta Miseviciene, Sean Redmond, Amanda Masterson, Hassan Slimi, Claire Beakhurst, Shauna Campbell, Grazina Pociute, Bobbi Hickey, Ciaran and Caoimhe Drennan, Sujan Ghimire, Darren Farrelly, Glen Cole, and 19 Rooms, Malta.

The Grafton Barber is a Proud Supporter of World Barber Day.